Praise for
Hunger in the Heartland

"This is a great guide to ways that those in the heartland and beyond can reach out to people in their communities who are struggling to put food on the table. The stories are compelling, and this guide suggests lots of practical ways to help."

—Rev. David Beckmann, President, Bread for the World

"Deb Engle and Rachel Quinn have written an outstanding resource guide not only for the heartland, but for any local communities where an interested individual or small group could ask the four questions lifted up in the guide: to find out what's already being done, to help, to see what's not being done and to do something about it. Engle and Quinn have written this guide by telling stories of folks who saw something that needed to be done in their community to feed the hungry and who found a way to get it done."

—Ambassador Tony Hall, President, Alliance to End Hunger,
Author of *Changing the Face of Hunger*

"What could be more embarrassing than hunger in the midst of the heartland—the world's breadbasket? But it's true—hunger does exist in the heartland and beyond, and as followers of Jesus we have a mandate to learn and to act. Engle and Quinn's *Hunger in the Heartland* resource guide has many helpful ways and resources to get started on alleviating hunger in your community. This guide is a good first step in ministering to 'the least of these' and, therefore, ministering to Jesus."

—Rich Pleva, Conference Minister, United Church of Christ in Iowa

"*Hunger in the Heartland* is a helpful resource for congregations and communities that seek to alleviate hunger in their local context. With stories, background information and clear suggestions for action, this guide persuasively demonstrates the need for the partnership between local efforts and the government assistance that is essential to effectively addressing the needs of those who live nutritionally insufficient lives. I recommend this resource to any and all who are willing to join the effort to make sure that those who are hungry will be fed."

—Rev. Michael L. Burk, Bishop, Southeastern Iowa Synod

"Food insecurity is typically a hidden problem in the heartland, which in turn causes a lack of awareness so that problems of academic performance, energy and nutrition go unattended. Engle and Quinn have not only lifted up issues that are faced in the heartland, they show folks how, in their own communities, they can address the hunger issues through grassroots partnering, community networking and organizing. Together we can work toward ending hunger in every community by each of us working in our own community to alleviate hunger there. *Hunger in the Heartland* is a great resource that gives people the helpful steps and resources they need to alleviate hunger where they live, work and play."

—Andy Bradley, Governor, Northeast Iowa District of Kiwanis International (2013-2014), Executive Vice President, Goodwill Industries, Inc.

"Hunger—especially childhood hunger—continues to be an embarrassment in a part of the U.S. that prides itself on feeding the world. When one in five of our children doesn't know where their next meal will come from—and when their families count on the school for food during the week and BackPack Program supplements on the weekend—we need to applaud compassionate writers like Engle and Quinn to help us make a difference in our communities. I highly endorse what they have accomplished in *Hunger in the Heartland*, and I hope it will receive the widespread coverage it deserves."

—Alan Scarfe, Bishop, Episcopal Diocese of Iowa

Hunger
in the
Heartland

*A Resource Guide
for Alleviating Hunger in Your Community,
No Matter Where You Live*

Debra Landwehr Engle
and Rachel Vogel Quinn

First GoldenTree Communications Edition
October 2014
© 2014 by Debra Landwehr Engle and Rachel Vogel Quinn

Cover design: Larrison Seidle
Cover photo: Anita Poeppel, Broad Branch Farm

Printed in the United States of America

ISBN: 9780978588311 soft cover
GoldenTree Communications, LLC
Winterset, Iowa
www.goldentreeco.com

To Don and Joyce Frevert,
in honor of their generosity and community
involvement. Together, they inspired countless others
to give the best of themselves for a better world.

Table of Contents

Foreword   1

Introduction   4

Hunger and Nutrition

Growing Up Hungry   8

The Food on Your Back   15

High School Hunger   20

The Role of Food Pantries   22

The Face of Hunger

SNAP: Myth vs. Reality   30

Feed Iowa First   34

Hidden Hunger: America's Veterans   37

Grocery Shopping 101   40

Reaching Out to the Elderly   43

The ABCs of Alleviating Hunger

Learning About Food ASAP   48

From the Farm to the School   54

Driving Away Hunger: Teens Take Charge   57

Farming for the Community   62

Rescuing Food and Land

Table to Table   68

Plant Your Parking   73

Alleviating Hunger, One Deer at a Time   76

The Great Pork Giveaway   80

Set Free   82

Spreading the Love   86

Bringing It All Together

Growing Faith   91

A Land to Call Home   98

Starting the Conversation   106

The Commitment of a Lifetime   111

15 Things You Can Do in the Next Hour   113

Discussion Questions   114

Thank You   118

Acknowledgments   121

Foreword

In 2007 I chaired a planning team assigned to organize a national symposium for the Alliance for Faith, Science, and Technology, part of the Evangelical Lutheran Church in America (ELCA). We were charged with focusing on a scientific issue and discovering how it was connected to our faith.

Since we're housed in the Midwest with lots of food resources—Iowa State University being one of them—our team decided the scientific issue should be food. We called the symposium "Food & Faith: Making the Connection." At the end of the symposium, these were the closing words:

> *You've heard about the scientific issues around food. You've learned how food is connected to your faith. Now what are you going to do about it when you get home?"*

When I asked myself that question, I decided I needed to form a small group, which I named "Food & Faith: A Call to Action." And so began a journey aligned with the United Nations' call for a global commitment to alleviate childhood hunger by 2015. The motto, "Global Goals...Local Solutions," tells the story: Do whatever you can, wherever you are.

It's hard to get one's head around alleviating all the childhood hunger in the world if we can't alleviate it right in our own community. In my area, one in five children is food-insecure. Seventy percent of the children in the Des Moines public school district where I live qualify for free or reduced-price lunches. In a state where 86 percent of the land is used for agriculture, we still have hungry children.

I discovered these things by reading, listening and attending informative meetings like the Iowa Hunger Summit and the World Food Prize's Borlaug Dialogues. As I learned, my passion grew. I invited a small group of people to join me in alleviating childhood hunger—not in the world, but right here at home. Here where we know folks, where our areas of influence exist, where surely we can make a difference.

Our group, the Coalition in Support of Hungry Children, started organizing annual conferences called Hope for the Hungry. These events bring together individuals in the Des Moines metro area with an interest in hunger issues to share ideas and best practices. Over the past few years, they have been attended by hundreds of people. Each conference focuses on practical applications, sending participants home with action steps and ideas they can implement right away.

Then, in December 2012, I had an inspiration, which turned into an email to author Deb Engle. "I have a crazy idea," I told her. "Have you ever thought about writing a sequel to *Grace from the Garden*?" That book, written by Deb several years ago, tells the stories of people across the country who are building their communities through gardening.

My email continued, "In our work with the Coalition in Support of Hungry Children to alleviate childhood hunger in greater Des Moines, we've learned about lots of folks who are doing exciting things to feed hungry people. You could write a book about these local efforts."

Deb's immediate reply? "Actually, I was thinking along those lines just this weekend. It's been 10 years since I wrote *Grace from the Garden*, and I was wondering if I should write a sequel."

And so began an exciting, scary, wonderful journey with a simple beginning—something we thought was going to be small but with a mighty message.

To tell this story—the story of folks who are food-insecure and the grassroots efforts to help—Tom Sawyer, filmmaker, and Deb, interviewer and author, created a documentary to inspire and inform viewers about hunger in the heartland.

As a companion to the documentary, this resource guide—a collaboration between Deb and writer Rachel Vogel Quinn—expands the story. Step by step, it provides direction to folks who want to make a difference in hungry people's lives.

That's what we all can do, if we just start where we are—if we just ask some simple questions:

What's already being done here?

How can I help?

What isn't being done that needs to be done?

What do I need to do to see that it happens?

It really is very easy, whether you take action as an individual or put together a small group of friends, fellow congregational members, or your service club companions. There's only one thing you need: To become passionate about alleviating childhood hunger in your community. Everything else will follow. *Hunger in the Heartland* will show you the way.

—Rev. Diana J. Sickles
June, 2014

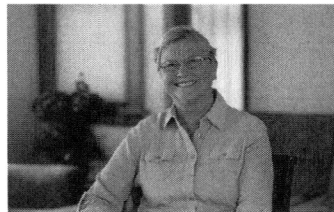

Introduction

"There should be no hunger in Iowa."

That statement, or some facsimile of it, has been voiced by virtually every person we've interviewed for this resource guide and the accompanying *Hunger in the Heartland* documentary.

Typically, the statement is made flat out, with no room for doubt or equivocation. The message is clear: There should be no hunger anywhere in this country or on this planet. But in Iowa? The state that helps feed the rest of the world? Maybe more than anywhere else, hunger in the heartland makes no sense logically or morally.

Iowa, after all, is about the land and the sustenance it produces. George Washington Carver is part of Iowa's agricultural tradition, along with Norman Borlaug, Henry Wallace, John Deere, the Leopold Center and the World Food Prize.

This is a salt-of-the-earth place, where the state's GNP is tied to agriculture. Yet here are the sobering statistics:

According to **feedingamerica.org**, more than 50 million people in the United States are hungry, including more than one in five children. Iowa mirrors the national statistics, with one in eight being food insecure (unsure where their next meal will come from). One in five children doesn't have enough to eat. More than 40 percent of Iowa's children qualify for free and reduced-price school lunches.

Iowa, though, is a microcosm of the U.S. for another reason. As Angie Tagtow, co-founder of the Iowa Food Systems Council, says, this is a place with a long tradition of neighbors helping one another. That's why, in addition to state and federal programs to help the hungry, Iowa has an active network of grassroots programs and committed individuals.

Matt Russell, state food policy project coordinator at the Drake University Agricultural Law Center, points out that these localized programs can't begin to replace the federal Supplemental Nutritional Assistance Program (SNAP). But they do several important things:

They fill in the gaps, making food available to people who need emergency help or are not on SNAP. They get local citizens involved. They shine a light on hunger and help educate communities about the hidden need. They raise the overall awareness of nutrition and wellness. And they can, in some cases, grow into larger programs that have a more widespread impact.

Community gardens, for instance, started with guerilla gardeners in a few cities across the U.S. in the 1970s and have since inspired a highly organized and visible movement that enriches neighborhoods while helping feed the hungry.

Feeding America's BackPack Program *(see page 15)* began with the simple idea of giving food-insecure kids something nutritious to eat on weekends during the school year. Now nearly 230,000 children across the country are served by this program every year.

And a pilot program—one that started small—incentivized SNAP participants to use their benefits to purchase fresh produce at farmer's markets. The data showed that the program helped change the buying habits of those SNAP recipients. Based on that success, it's now part of the U.S. Farm Bill, which includes the federal food assistance program.

From churches to schools to concerned individuals, more solutions to hunger are sprouting up every day to meet that growing need. That's what this book is about. It's about how people are helping, specifically what they're doing and how you can replicate their work or use it as a jumping-off point for your own idea.

In short, this book addresses the basics of hunger so you can do something about the issue in your own community. Even though the information is gleaned from Iowa, the same ideas will work anywhere. That's why it's a resource guide, including websites and contact information for many of the people featured. They all are willing to share their ideas to help you help the hungry.

The thing is, the hungry may be your neighbors, folks at your church or kids at your children's school. And one day, they could be you, since so many hunger issues are created by divorce, health issues or unexpected job loss.

So instead of shaking our heads in hopelessness or shame, we can simply take action. Do one thing. There are hundreds of examples and ideas in this book, and some of them are as simple as making a phone call or digging in the dirt.

There's no doubt that food is a political issue. It's an issue of poverty, access and discrimination. But underneath all of that, food is a basic need. And especially for children and the elderly, it's a health issue that won't wait for political debates to be resolved. For the child whose school lunch is the only real meal of the day or the homebound senior citizen who lives in a rural area where the nearest grocery store is 30 miles away, alleviating hunger is about taking action today.

That's why this book is about the solution rather than the problem. And more specifically, the solution that lies within your backyard, your school, your church, your grocery store, your food pantry. The solution doesn't have to be large or complicated or expensive. As the citizens in this book demonstrate, it all starts with a desire as basic as food itself: the desire to help another human being.

—Debra Landwehr Engle

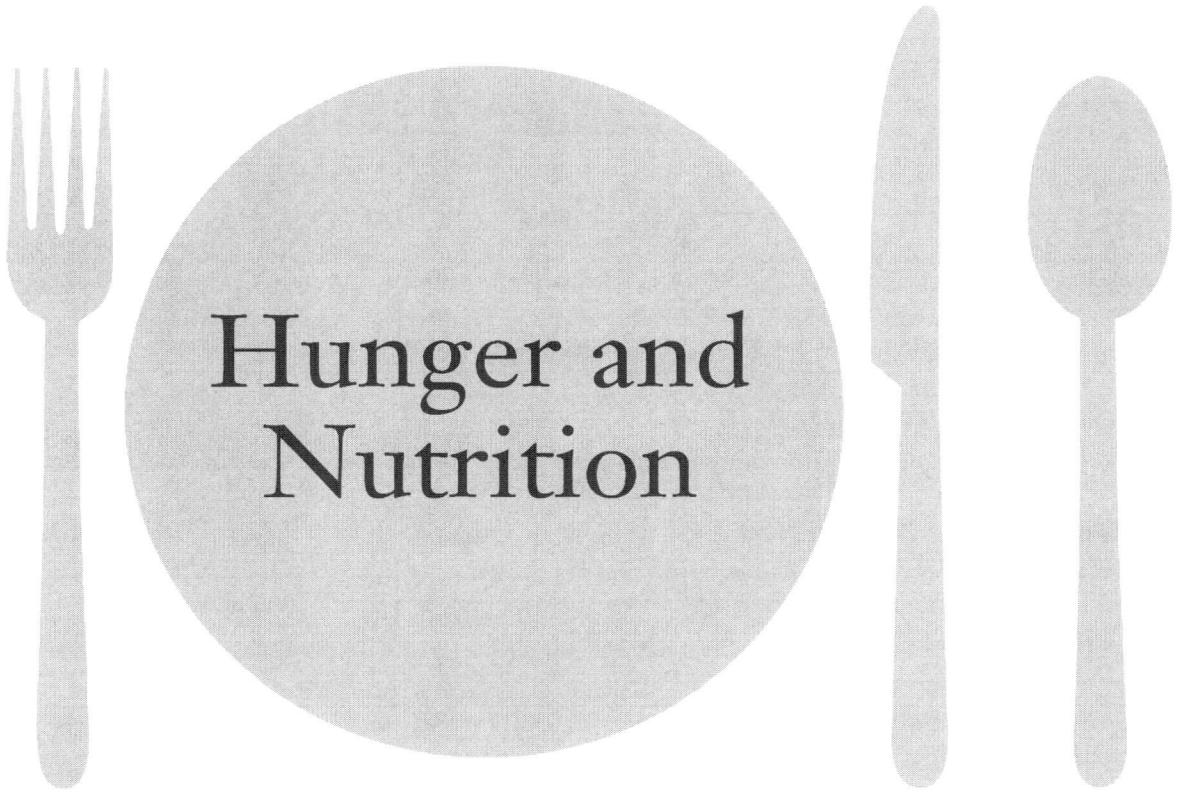

Hunger and Nutrition

Growing Up Hungry

Hunger may have the most devastating effects on children, whose entire lives can be affected by what they eat early on. Here, from a medical perspective, is a look at the pressing issues around hunger and kids.

We talked with Dr. David Spreadbury, Ph.D., professor emeritus of nutrition at Des Moines University, about the long-term impact of poor nutrition on kids—and why a home-cooked meal could help turn things around.

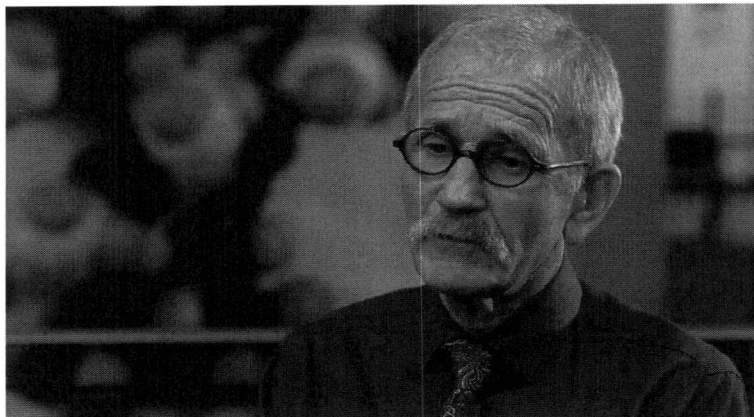

Dr. Spreadbury, professor emeritus of nutrition at Des Moines University.

Q. You've been teaching at Des Moines University for 36 years. What changes have you seen in hunger issues over that time?
A. It seems to me that there is a greater need now. Things appear to have gotten much worse over the past four or five years since the economic downturn. I hear pediatricians say that they're now seeing more malnourished children than at any time since the Great Depression.

Q. What's the impact of nutrition on children, beginning with infants?
A. Adequate nutrition is very important right from the beginning of pregnancy. For example, if a woman has too low an intake of folate during the first month of pregnancy, she's at a much higher risk of giving birth to a neural tube baby with spina bifida or a similar condition. It's critical that first month when a woman may not even know she's pregnant, and that carries on throughout pregnancy.

Research over the last 20 or 30 years shows that if anything impairs growth during pregnancy, that individual is at greater risk for a number of diseases, even as an adult. Being born small for one's gestational age is a great disadvantage, and there's no catching up from it.

Physiologically, the growth of these children is restricted and they have smaller body size than they should for their age. Brain development can be affected. Again, many of those effects are not remediable. You can't catch up afterward. Therefore you're impaired throughout life.

Q. Are there other effects of poor nutrition on children?
A. A child can be more susceptible to infectious disease. Or, if children have a disease, it could last longer because their immune system is impaired by

inadequate nutrition. They can be pre-programmed for higher risk for noncommunicable diseases in adulthood, such as diabetes, coronary heart disease and osteoporosis.

Because of the higher risk of disease, they're going to consume a higher portion of the health care budget. It's in our economic self-interest to make sure people have a good start in life and remain healthy as long as possible.

Q. How does poor nutrition impact children's performance in school?
A. There's good evidence that learning is more difficult if the brain is not developing normally. A malnourished child is at much greater risk of having to repeat a year in school. That handicap stays with them throughout their school years. Hungry adolescents are more aggressive, have more anxiety and have greater difficulty paying attention. They're not able

to learn adequately. Therefore their income as adults is impacted, perpetuating poverty and malnutrition.

Q. The rate of obesity among children is growing. Are obesity and malnutrition linked?
A. We have 9 million obese and overweight individuals in this country and 14 million hungry individuals. It seems paradoxical. How can those two co-exist? We have to differentiate between being hungry and being malnourished.

For example, if you're hungry, you could eat a donut and you'll no longer feel hungry, but you will have taken in very few nutrients. At the same time, you could eat a slice of whole wheat bread and peanut butter. You'll no longer be hungry, but you will have taken in a significant number of nutrients. So you can be obese and malnourished at the same time. Obesity is an indicator that you've taken in

too many calories. It does not mean that you've taken in an adequate number of nutrients.

We require over 40 essential nutrients per day in our diet. Those are nutrients the body simply can't synthesize, so we must get them from our diet. But our primary need is for calories. If we get our calories from the wrong source—from foods with few nutrients, like pop and sugar and so forth—we can be malnourished. But we're taking in more than adequate calories, so we can become obese.

Q. What happens if we don't get those 40 essential nutrients?
A. In our society, we don't very often see real vitamin or mineral deficiencies—not in the classic sense we saw a hundred years ago. But what we do see is inadequate intake of a number of these essential vitamins and minerals, and the effects are less easy to spot. There's no doubt they will impair a

person's ability to function, and for their brains to function at an optimum level.

Q. How can we be sure children are getting the right nutrients?
A. The plan for a good diet is encapsulated in the USDA's My Plate **[www.choosemyplate. gov]**, which indicates that a healthy diet should be three-quarters fruits, vegetables and whole grains, and the rest protein sources. Eighty-five percent of grains consumed in this country are highly refined grains, which are much less nutritious than whole grains. One good place to start is to incorporate whole grains as much as possible.

We have been singularly un-successful in the last 25 years in encouraging people to eat more fruits and vegetables. The number of servings per day hasn't gone up. Part of that is you have to show people how to prepare them.

Fewer and fewer people are preparing their own food. It seems a natural progression. We used to make our own clothes, build our own houses. But we're handing over food preparation to other people now.

Q. What's the impact of handing over food preparation to others?
A. Research has shown that home-prepared food tends to be more nutritious. It contains more of the nutrients we need every day than commercially prepared or fast food or restaurant food. It tends to be cheaper as well.

Q. Why aren't people cooking these days?
A. Food preparation is a major business. The majority of the food eaten now is prepared by other people: commercially prepared food, fast food, restaurants, packaged food. So much of a person's cooking now is in the microwave. Probably the microwave has changed food preparation in the U.S.

more than any other single thing. These foods tend to be poorer nutritionally. We have to try to get back to the basics and prepare some of our food ourselves.

Food preparation is not taught in schools like it used to be. Parents tend to not pass it along to their children because they themselves do not cook or are unable to cook because they don't know how.

Fast food is very carefully designed to be so tasty that it's irresistible. We've gotten so clever at manipulating tastes through taste chemists, who can give people an orgasm in the mouth just by tasting things. If you're in the food business, your ultimate objective is to get people to buy and consume more of it. There are 4,000 calories per person released into the market every day. That's twice as much as the average person needs, so you have to try to sell it somehow. How do you stay in business? You

Cooking Up Better Health

According to Dr. Spreadbury, only 25 percent of medical schools in the U.S. teach classes in nutrition, which means many health professionals can't provide guidance to their patients on the importance of healthy eating.

Dr. Spreadbury lobbied for a teaching kitchen at Des Moines University for a specific reason: "What we try to do is encourage students to look at their own diets and consider how healthy they are. We've been very successful in getting a lot of students to change the way they eat."

Here are a few tips from his teaching kitchen to help your own families and those in your community.

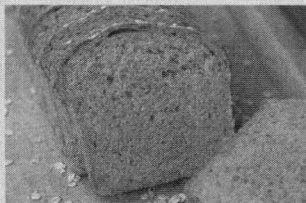

If you do one thing, just move to whole grains. "When you buy a loaf of bread," Dr. Spreadbury says, "it should not be multigrain—it has to say 100 percent whole wheat. When you buy rice, buy whole grain rice. Whole grain cereals are so much more nutritionally complete than refined cereal. That's a fairly easy thing to do. Most people find they like the taste of the whole grain more than the old one."

Introduce more vegetables in your diet. "Try to incorporate vegetables once a week, then twice a week," Dr. Spreadbury says. "A lot of it's in the preparation." To prove the point, he serves his students Brussels sprouts, which typically elicit collective groans at first. "We sauté frozen Brussels sprouts in a little bit of butter for thirty minutes. The sugars in the sprouts caramelize and become delicious and nutty. We convert haters to addicts in that one tasting." The key? It has to taste good. But eating healthy doesn't have to be expensive. "You can buy a good bag of Brussels sprouts for just over a dollar," he says.

Keep it simple. Another favorite in the teaching kitchen is oven-roasted root vegetables, Dr. Spreadbury says. "Beets and carrots and parsnips and rutabagas and kohlrabi—all sorts of exotic things. People love them because they're so tasty." Again, simple preparation is key. "You don't boil these things or you destroy them," he says. "Water and vegetables are enemies. Use as little water as possible. Sauté them or roast them."

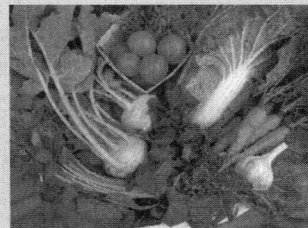

either charge more for it or get people to eat more of it.

Q. How do you teach nutrition to your students?
A. We teach nutrition in the curriculum here to the medical students, the physician assistant students and the podiatry students. You can teach nutrition in a couple of ways: via chemistry, which is intracellular—or you can relate it to food because, in my book, nutrition is what you put on your plate. We have to have those 40 essential vitamins and minerals.

What we try to do is encourage students to look at their own diets and consider how healthy they are. We've been very successful in getting a lot of students to change the way they eat. That's music to my ears. The incorporation of the teaching kitchen is an extension of this. We will show you how to prepare it. That's the stage we're at now.

I honestly believe that if we

Dr. Spreadbury's Butternut Squash Chili

This is one of several recipes that have turned doubters into vegetable lovers in classes at Des Moines University.

1 medium butternut squash peeled, seeded and cubed into
   ½-inch pieces
1 large onion, chopped
2 cloves garlic, chopped
½ to 1 whole jalapeno, finely chopped
1 red or green pepper, chopped
A few shakes of Tabasco, chipotle flavor
1 tablespoon chili powder
1 teaspoon ground cumin
1 16-ounce can tomato sauce
1 16-ounce can Bush's pinto beans, drained
1 16-ounce can black beans, drained
2 tablespoons canola oil
   Grated cheddar or vegan cheese for garnish
   (optional)

1. In a large pan, sauté the onion in canola oil for a few minutes on medium high until beginning to brown. Add the squash, jalapeno, pepper and garlic together with the spices and Tabasco, and sauté with a lid on. Stir occasionally until the squash begins to soften.

2. Add the beans and tomato sauce, and bring to a simmer. Transfer to a slow cooker; set on low and cook for several hours. Garnish with cheese if desired.

can get an individual to change their own lifestyle, particularly as a physician, they're more likely to be an advocate with their patients, and they'll have much higher credibility with their patients if they're practicing good nutrition themselves. This is true particularly of pediatricians, who are more prevention-oriented than other physicians. If a physician isn't tuned in to what their patients are eating and doesn't mention it, the message to the patient is that it's not important.

Q. You have a fully equipped teaching kitchen on campus. What do you hope to accomplish by teaching your students how to cook?
A. My primary target is that they'll pay attention to their own diets and then make some improvements, which creates a multiplier effect. When they have a patient with diabetes or coronary heart disease, they'll emphasize to that patient how important it is to eat the appropriate diet.

It's been shown by Dr. Dean Ornish and others that people with advanced coronary heart disease can reverse the process completely if they change their diet sufficiently, and if we encourage them to exercise and learn meditation techniques to reduce stress. What we don't know is how to persuade people to make those changes. That's where we come in. If we get students convinced that nutrition is important, they'll incorporate it in their practices and be agents for change.

Q. Will you offer cooking classes off campus as well?
A. We're expanding this to the outside community. We're doing this tentatively because we have restricted resources and none of us are professionally trained chefs. We're just learning on the job.

I fantasize that we would expand our teaching kitchen here to a fully equipped vehicle with a teaching kitchen in it. This could be taken around Iowa to show people how to prepare healthy food and what it tastes like. Can you imagine at the Iowa State Fair competing with Twinkies on a stick, showing that healthy food can taste good?

Q. Why is it important to help the hungry?
A. I think one of the hallmarks of any advanced society is that it's able to take care of its disadvantaged. So much of life is where we were born, adequate childhood nutrition, etc. The gap between the haves and have-nots in our society is widening. And there's a very narrow gap sometimes as far as whether we make it or we don't. I don't think we should look at society purely in terms of how much wealth it generates, but also how well it looks after our impoverished individuals.

How Can Obesity and Hunger Co-exist?

For anyone who grew up seeing ads about starving children in other parts of the world, hunger equals emaciation, with distended bellies, gaunt faces and hollow eyes. That's part of the reason why hunger in America is such a hidden problem, because hunger here often looks 180 degrees opposite of famine. It often looks like obesity.

As Dr. David Spreadbury says, "Obesity is an indicator that you've taken in too many calories. It does not mean that you've taken in an adequate number of nutrients."

Here's a look at obesity and health by the numbers.

In 1980, percentage of U.S. children ages 6 to 11 who were obese: **7**

In 2012, percentage of U.S. children ages 6 to 11 who were obese: **18**

In 1980, percentage of U.S. adolescents ages 12 to 19 who were obese: **5**

In 2012, percentage of U.S. adolescents ages 12 to 19 who were obese: **21**

In 2012, percentage of U.S. children and adolescents who were overweight or obese: **More than 33**

Among obese children ages 5 to 17, percentage with at least one risk factor (such as high cholesterol or high blood pressure) for cardiovascular disease: **70**

Long-term health risks for children and adolescents who are obese: **Heart disease, type 2 diabetes, stroke, cancer, osteoarthritis**

Types of cancer for which overweight and obese people have an increased risk long-term: **Breast, colon, endometrium, esophagus, kidney, pancreas, gall bladder, thyroid, ovary, cervix and prostate, plus multiple myeloma and Hodgkin's lymphoma**

Number of times a week of eating fast food required to increase risk for weight gain, overweight and obesity: **One or more**

Average amount of full-calorie soda consumed daily by U.S. male adolescents ages 12 to 19: **22 oz.**

Average amount of milk consumed daily by U.S. male adolescents ages 12 to 19: **10 oz.**

Behaviors linked to eating a healthy breakfast: **Improved cognitive function (especially memory), reduced absenteeism, improved mood**

Percentage of medical schools in the U.S. that offer nutrition education to future health professionals: **25**

Increase in hospitalizations of obese children and youths between 1999 and 2005: **Nearly double**

Total cost for children and youths with obesity-related hospitalizations in 2001: **$125.9 million**

Total cost for children and youths with obesity-related hospitalizations in 2005: **$237.6 million**

By 2030, percentage of U.S. adults projected to be obese: **50**

Percentage of Americans with diabetes: **8.3 (nearly 26 million children and adults)**

By 2030, projected medical costs associated with treating preventable obesity-related diseases: **$66 billion per year**

By 2030, projected annual loss in economic productivity: **Between $390 billion and $580 billion**

Sources: Centers for Disease Control and Prevention at cdc.gov, American Diabetes Association

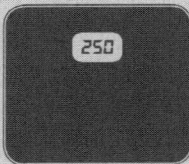

Q. What's the difference between "overweight" and "obese"?

A. According to the Centers for Disease Control and Prevention, "Overweight is defined as having excess body weight for a particular height from fat, muscle, bone, water or a combination of these factors. Obesity is defined as having excess body fat."

The Food on Your Back

For food-insecure children, a national BackPack Program comes to the rescue during one of the most difficult times of the week.

It's Monday morning, and school nurses across the U.S. are experiencing one of their busiest times of the week. Children are complaining of headaches and stomachaches—not because of what they've eaten, but because they haven't eaten at all.

In many of the nation's food-insecure families, children may go an entire weekend without a real meal. To address the problem, Feeding America's Back-Pack Program aims to lessen the consequences of hunger in elementary schools by providing low-resource children with easy-to-prepare foods over the weekend.

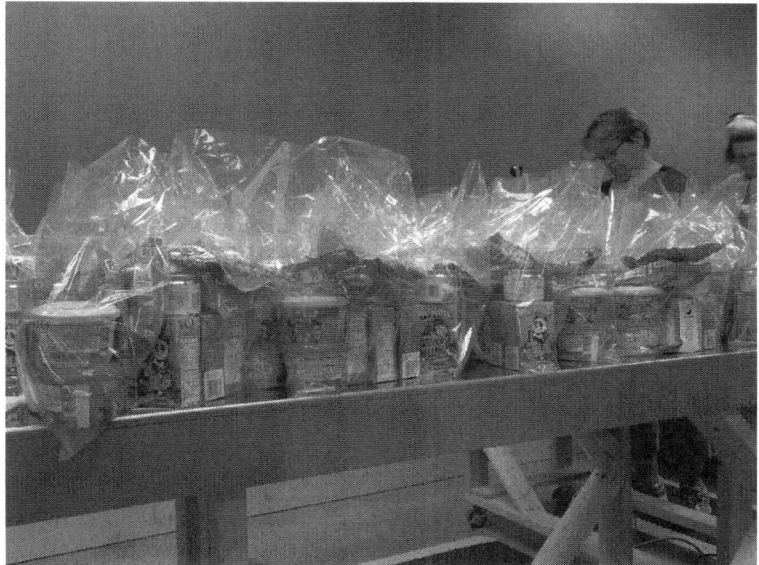

The back-to-school season is a busy time for Food Bank for the Heartland. In August, volunteers come to the warehouse to pack weekend meals into clear sacks, which can be slipped into backpacks.

The program began in Little Rock, Arkansas, in 1999, when a school nurse recognized the pattern in the Monday morning office visits: The kids had hardly eaten on Saturday and Sunday.

Now the BackPack Program serves more than 230,000 elementary schoolchildren nationwide. In Iowa, five food banks serve hungry children in schools across the state.

"Our kids are in a population that is among the most vulnerable," says Matt Unger, program manager at the Food Bank of Iowa, which serves 42 counties in the central portion of the state. "We feel a responsibility to step up and do something."

"Our programs, like the BackPack Program, fill the gap of child hunger," says Michelle Sause, child hunger program manager at Food Bank for the Heartland, which serves 93 counties in Nebraska and western Iowa. "We have wonderful agency partners, such as food pantries, but they are not necessarily geared toward children."

In Iowa, the number of children who receive backpacks is soaring. Both the Food Bank of weekend meals for 4,500 children at 113 schools. But it still isn't enough. "We're just a small Band-Aid on feeding these hungry kids over the weekend," says Unger.

Backpack Blessing

Although it's called the BackPack Program, the food is usually packed in grocery sacks or clear plastic bags, which can be quietly slipped into backpacks during recess or lunch to maintain confidentiality. The bags contain two breakfasts, two lunches and a snack for the weekend, along with milk and juice *(see sidebar, left)*.

All the items are shelf-stable, meaning they don't require refrigeration. The food is also ready to eat without any preparation. "Even little kids can maneuver and access it without using a microwave," says Sause.

At the Food Bank of Iowa, all the food for the BackPack Program is purchased fresh and brand new. At first, the organization experimented with food drives, but they often received sugary snacks and food with early expiration dates. They also ended up with such a variety of foods that they never could fill even one school's order with the same items.

Although the program is the Food Bank of Iowa's most expensive, it is funded fully through donations. For less than $4 a week, a donor can feed one child over the weekend.

Four times a year, the students in the Food

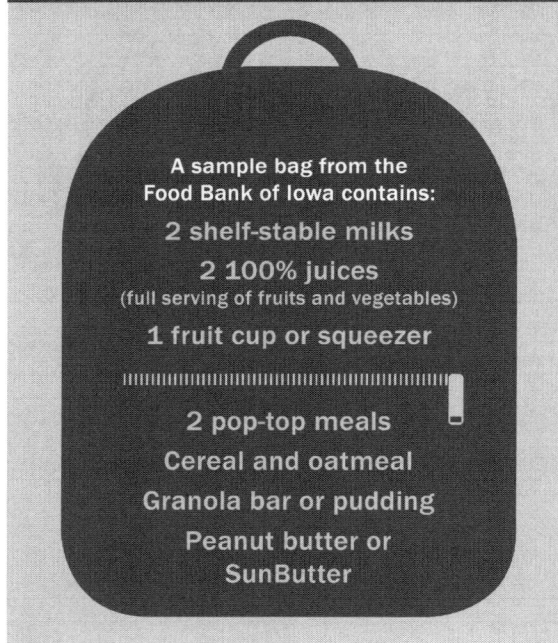

Iowa and Food Bank for the Heartland have doubled the number of students they serve in the last year.

The Food Bank of Iowa alone provides

Bank of Iowa's BackPack Program and the Northeast Iowa Food Bank's BackPack Program receive $5 coupons for sliced or shaved ham, enough for about one pound from the meat counter.

The coupons are provided by the Deb and Jeff Hansen Foundation, founders of Iowa Select Farms, the state's largest pork producer.

The foundation chose ham because it is a nutrient-dense, lean protein that promotes growth and development. *(For more on the Deb and Jeff Hansen Foundation, see page 80).*

The food banks leave it up to school administrators to decide what day they distribute.

Mostly, though, the kids eat the food over Saturday and Sunday, leaving them healthy and ready for school on Monday.

"These kids are so excited on Fridays to bring their sacks home," says Unger.

Happy Friday

At no cost to the schools or families, the Back-Pack Program is a godsend to the students participating. Most often, food banks decide how many children to serve at each school based on a percentage of students receiving free and reduced-price meals through the National School Lunch Program, School

Piggyback on the BackPack Program

Whether you want to join the national BackPack Program or start something similar on your own, keep these tips from Matt Unger and Michelle Sause in mind.

Start small. To keep costs in check, Unger suggests getting your model and logistics down before you start growing the BackPack Program.

Find a champion. Seek out community partners among corporations, service clubs and individuals. The Food Bank of Iowa, for example, gets support from Variety the Children's Charity, Prairie Meadows, Nationwide and the John Deere Foundation.

Make it a community program. Getting local citizens on board is essential. You'll need volunteers to help pack bags and donors to send checks. "It spreads like wildfire once folks know about it," says Unger.

Build relationships. To reach schools in small towns, it's best to know someone. "In our rural communities, they can feel like it's the big city coming in to fix everything," says Sause. To prevent that, Food Bank for the Heartland focuses on cultivating personal relationships with all their schools.

Breakfast Program and the Afterschool Care Snack Program.

Sause says she is confident that low-resource children are receiving two good meals each school day through these programs. Food Bank for the Heartland picks up the slack.

Although the number of free and re-duced-price lunches provides a guideline, the schools get to decide which students are selected for the program, since they know the students best. The food bank hands out a guide to principals, teachers, nurses and cafeteria staff, advising them how to recognize the signs of child hunger.

Schools must be vigilant in finding the hungry children, despite their income status. "There are a lot of families that fall in that gap where they may not receive free and reduced-price lunch or SNAP because a parent got a 50-cent raise that knocked them off benefits," says Sause. The BackPack Program allows schools to serve those children who may not qualify on paper but still have a need.

At Lamoni Elementary, served by the Food Bank of Iowa, the staff uses the guidelines to select between 35 and 40 kids each year. A local church stores the food and helps pack and deliver the bags every week.

The site coordinator slips the sacks into backpacks over recess, to make sure no child is

How You Can Help

Volunteer. Contact your local food bank to see if they need help packing bags each month.

Donate money. For less than $4 a week, you can provide a weekend's worth of food for a hungry child.

Become a community partner. See if your organization is interested in joining forces with an elementary school to pack bags and deliver food. If not, one or two individuals can do it on their own.

Involve your school. If your local school doesn't participate, find out if there is a need, even for a few students. Then contact your local food bank for details on the application process.

teased. Still, not all kids are embarrassed by the program; most are just happy about the food.

When Stacy Jones, site coordinator for Lamoni, walks down the hall at the end of the week, she often is greeted by shouts of "Yay!" and "It's Friday! We get our backpacks!"

Working Together

About 75 percent of the Food Bank of Iowa's schools have a community partner—such as a church, local business, Rotary Club or hospi-tal—that picks up the boxes, gathers volunteers to pack food into sacks and delivers the sacks to the school each week. For two days a month, the Food Bank invites volunteers to their warehouse to pack bags for local schools and those without community partners.

Food Bank for the Heartland, which used to get already-packed bags from another food bank, now hand-packs 90 percent of their food.

Student Success: You Are What You Eat

Studies show that nutrition is correlated with academic performance, which means kids in the BackPack Program get the support to do their best in school.

- Hunger is associated with lower grades, more absences, repeating a grade and an inability to focus.
- Students who skip breakfast are less alert and have more difficulty solving problems.
- A lack of nutritious food—especially fruits, vegetables or dairy products—is associated with lower grades.
- A lack of certain vitamins and minerals is related to lower grades and more absences and tardiness.

Source: Centers for Disease Control and Prevention

The food in those sacks—just four meals and a snack—can go a long way in improving children's lives and their school performance. On surveys given each year, parents say their kids concentrate better because they're not as hungry. Attendance is better for the participating kids on Mondays and Fridays. Many studies show the link between a sufficient, nutritious diet and academic achievement.

"The program is giving them a chance to have a shot at coming to school on Monday and actually being able to get something out of school rather than just worrying about how bad they feel," says Unger.

But no one says it better than the kids themselves, who write down their thoughts about the food during the survey. A sampling of their comments:

"Thank you for BackPack. This is the best day of my life."

"Me and my family like this because it gives us food we need."

"It's a great idea to help families out. Thanks for the best food ever!"

FOR MORE DETAILS about the BackPack Program, visit **www.feedingamerica.org**. There you'll find the Food Bank Locator, which will help you identify BackPack programs in your community.

High School Hunger

The national BackPack Program focuses on elementary-age children, but older students are hungry, too. Perry High School is helping teens who fall into that gap.

Tami Valline, school counselor at Perry High School in Perry, Iowa, knew something was wrong when she started hearing kids say they didn't eat outside of school. Deciding to do something about it, Valline talked with her principal about the need for some kind of help inside the building.

When a classroom opened up, they began a school food pantry with the help of a retired English teacher, an at-risk associate and other school staff.

"We were worried about the weekends especially, when some of our parents might be working, out of town or just not around," Valline says about the decision to open a pantry. "We worried about what the students were eating—or if they were eating."

For a small school in a small town, Perry has a high number of students receiving free and reduced-price meals. Although the town has a food pantry, its distance from the school and some of the students' lack of transportation meant that teenagers weren't using it.

"When we got started, we were looking to fill

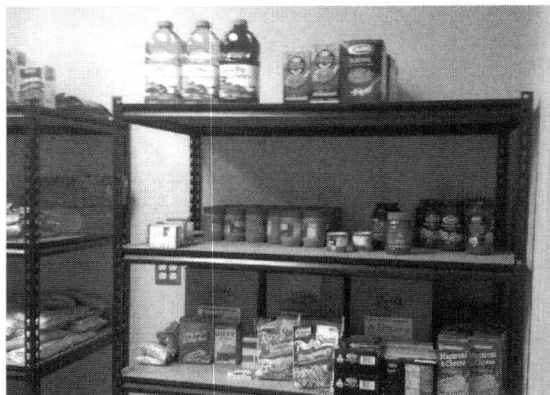

A few shelving units and lights were all it took to turn an unused room in Perry High School into a food pantry.

Photo: Jon Larson

that void of students who were falling through the cracks," she says.

Valline found that starting the pantry was much easier than she initially thought. A team put up some shelves, a few lights and a camera for security.

Donations started coming in from drives for food and personal care items at football games, as well as from citizens who dropped off checks. The city pantry also provides some food.

The pantry is open every day, all day, during

"ANY TIME IT FEELS THAT PEOPLE CARE ABOUT THEM, WANT THEM TO SUCCEED AND ARE WILLING TO GO ABOVE AND BEYOND TO MAKE SURE THEY HAVE WHAT THEY NEED, IT'S MORE LIKELY THEY ARE GOING TO PERFORM BETTER IN SCHOOL."

the school year and serves between two and six kids a week, many on a regular basis. There are no qualifications for who can use it or how often.

Students see one of the school counselors when they need food, and the adults either pack a backpack for them or take them to the pantry in a low-traffic area of the school to pick out what they want.

Valline says that some of the kids using the pantry live on their own or don't have much adult supervision.

They prefer simple items they can easily prepare, such as macaroni and cheese, hot dogs, tuna, cereal, canned fruit and vegetables and pasta.

"The kids who use it regularly are probably more connected to the school," says Valline. "Any time it feels that people care about them, want them to succeed and are willing to go above and beyond to make sure they have what they need, it's more likely they are going to perform better in school."

Starting a School Food Pantry

Tami Valline advises schools interested in setting up a pantry to jump in. The cost, she says, is less than you might think. Here are a few important tips:

- **Find local supporters,** such as a Rotary or Kiwanis Club. Talk to members of those service clubs in your community to help fund and organize the pantry.

- **Solicit nonperishable foods.** Since use of the pantry may be sporadic, canned and packaged foods with a long shelf life are best.

- **Promote healthy choices.** Encourage donors to consider nutrition as well as kids' preferences. Teens may love sugary snacks, but they need foods that will give them nutritive value.

- **Be patient.** Know that you are helping students, even if only a few need it. "Sometimes, we will have a whole week where it's not used at all, and that's fine," says Valline. "The kids know it's there when they need it."

The Role of Food Pantries

Forming a distribution system all across the country, these local outlets meet the rising need for emergency and supplemental assistance.

We talked with Bernadette Egger, on-site coordinator at Catholic Charities, St. Mary Family Center in Des Moines, Iowa, about the role of food pantries in alleviating hunger.

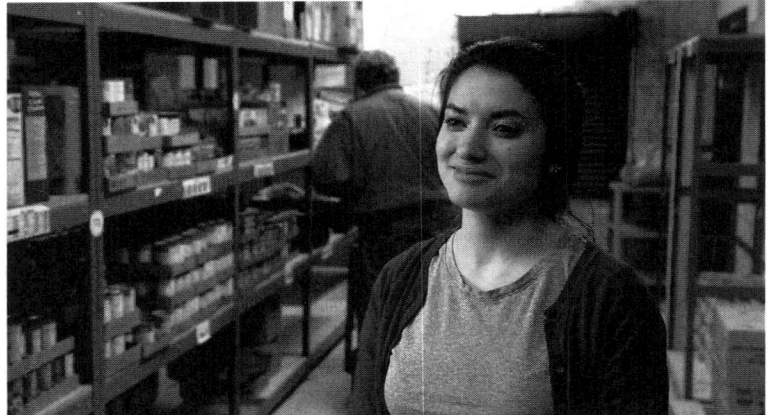

Bernadette Egger of St. Mary Family Center.

Q. Why is hunger important to you?
A. I think that when you think about all the things that affect people in different ways, hunger is one of those things that gets right in there and cuts you to the quick. In order to solve a lot of other problems, I think we need to start with feeding people.

Q. How many people does St. Mary's serve?
A. Every day, St. Mary's sees about 400 people walk in the door to use our food counter items. Every month, we see about 700 people use our emergency food boxes. The four-day emergency food box is through a partnership with the Des Moines Area Religious Council (DMARC) and **MovetheFood. org**. It goes by family size. It's a nutritionally balanced box that will last a particular number of family members for four days.

Q. When do people use emergency food boxes?
A. It could be absolutely anything. If you're using the emergency food box services, it could be something as simple as you broke your leg last month. You can't go to your job, and you end up spending more on medical bills and less on food, so you need the assistance. Maybe you work a seasonal job. If you're a painter, the winter months can be rough because you aren't able to paint outside, so you come in a little more to use those services.

Maybe you're expanding your family. Maybe you've got a child who needs a specific kind of formula. Formula is so expensive—we see this all the time. If you're putting more of your food budget toward formula for your child, it means less for the rest of the family. It's a lot easier to find food assistance than it is to find formula. Also, we see a lot of people moving to Iowa because it's a great place to live. But when you start from absolutely nothing, it's more important to spend that money on shelter, especially

"I WISH THAT THE PUBLIC KNEW HOW MUCH HUNGER AFFECTS EVERYONE IN THE FAMILY— EVERYBODY FROM THE NEWBORN BABY ON UP TO THE SENIOR CITIZENS."

during the winter, than it is to work on your food budget.

Q. Why is there such a demand for baby formula?
A. If you're a working mom, you're not going to be able to take the time off to breast-feed your baby, so you're going to need to have formula. The difficult part of providing formula for your children is that the price is so high, comparatively speaking. If your child happens to have any allergies, the price goes up and up and up. We expect people to do what's best for their newborn and for their family—to hold the job and to feed their children. That causes a lot of problems.

Q. What other challenges do you see in the winter?
A. One of our challenges is having something for everybody.

It's hard when you look at your cooler in the morning and you have four crates of milk, and you need to be open until 3:30 and could see 400 people come in. How do you make that last so it's worthwhile for the clients?

Q. How do you meet that need?
A. Luckily, we have a lot of

fantastic donors. We get support from DMARC and Movethe-Food network. We get support from the Food Bank of Iowa and from local businesses like Anderson Erickson Dairy, Hy-Vee and Panera Bread. Without that support, I honestly don't know how we'd keep going. With a lot of help, we make it work.

Q. Do small individual donations help?
A. I'd say there's no such thing as too little. A lot of people get in that thought process of, "If I

Food Bank/Food Pantry: What's the Difference?

In Iowa, the **food bank** serves as a warehouse and distribution center, accepting food donations from growers, packers, processors, manufacturers, wholesalers, brokers and retailers, as well as the USDA. The food bank distributes food to its network of food pantries and other community partners.

A **food pantry** is a local outlet that receives food from the food bank, along with other corporate and individual donations, and makes it available at locations around the community to individuals in need. Food pantries may be operated by churches, nonprofit organizations or others.

can't donate a ton of stuff, why bother? Why bother bringing in the extra zucchini from my garden?" Every little bit can definitely help somebody. In the summertime, we will ask local gardeners to please stop sticking zucchini in your friend's car and bring it down to the food pantry instead. Our clients are really excited to see that. They would rather eat healthy than eat macaroni and cheese out of a box.

Q. Is that a misconception about people who use pantries?

A. It's definitely a misconception that people would rather take home a boxed dinner instead of making zucchini bread or pasta or stuffed peppers—something like that. We definitely have a lot of clients who cook and would rather start from scratch than eat from a box.

Q. What other misconceptions do you see?

A. I think there's a misconception that food pantry clients are people who are not trying to pull themselves up from underneath the poverty line, that people use food pantries because it's easier than spending money at a grocery store.

We don't have income restrictions here, and when people find out, sometimes they're surprised. They wonder, "How do you know if someone really truly needs it?"

But the question I always ask them is, "If you did not need a food pantry, would you really come here to get the canned food items? If you weren't truly in need, would you really spend your gas and time to come here to get our canned goods and what we happen to be giving out over the counter?" The answer is no. If you did not need it, you would not use it.

Q. What do you want the public to know?

A. I wish the public knew how much hunger affects everyone in the family—everybody from the newborn baby on up to the senior citizens. Especially senior citizens. We have a lot of clients who are elderly, and they need as much resource as someone with four kids. If you're aging and have health problems, it's hard to find something to accommodate that. If you're a diabetic, you've got to look at your food choices a little more carefully. We try to support that in our clients.

Q. How many of your clients are employed?

A. About 85 percent of our clientele hold steady jobs and have steady income. That does not include our elderly population, nor does it include the homeless people we serve. About 85 percent have jobs, and it's still just not enough.

TO FIND A FOOD PANTRY NEAR YOU that accepts fresh produce, visit **www. ampleharvest.org**. You can search for food pantries in or near your zip code and see what days and times they accept donations.

Five Simple Ways to Support Your Local Food Pantry

1. Donate fresh produce.
As Bernadette Egger says, don't worry that your contribution is too small. If you're a gardener, plant extra and donate it. Every bit helps.

2. Donate your time.
Most food pantries need help with everything from stocking shelves to greeting clients as they come in. Again, don't underestimate the value of an hour or two of your time per week or month.

3. Initiate a food pantry drive in your church, company, book club, neighborhood group or other organization.
Be sure to coordinate with your local food pantry to see what kinds of food items they need most. Also, check on food safety considerations and the time of year they have the greatest need. For instance, they might appreciate a food drive during times of the year when pantries can be forgotten, such as January through May—after the holidays and before fresh produce is available.

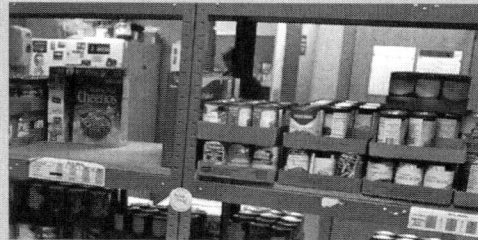

4. Donate money.
Food banks and food pantries often negotiate lower prices with wholesale distributors because they need such large quantities of food. As a result, they may be able to purchase a packaged food for a tenth of the price you'd pay, making your cash donation go much further. According to the Food Bank of Iowa, they can provide 4.5 meals for every $1 donation.

5. Spread the word about the important work food pantries do.
Use social media and other means to encourage friends to make a donation.

The Gift of Groceries

A Guide to Donating to Your Local Food Pantry

Too often, food pantries receive donations from the back of the shelf—unappetizing or expired items that the donors don't want. Next time you're considering a donation, take this list to the grocery store and buy brand-new items for the low-resource families served by your local pantry. Or give cash that your food pantry can use to buy what it needs most.

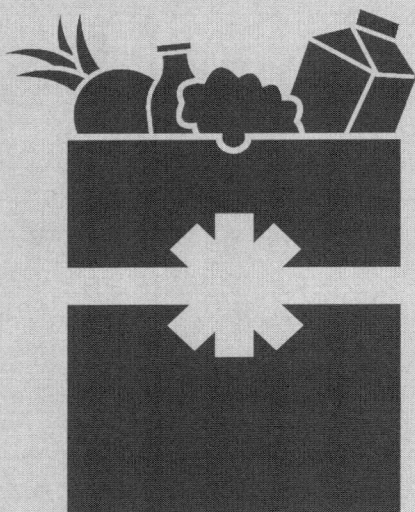

Call ahead.

The storage capabilities of every food pantry differ. Some have freezers and refrigerators, others only shelves. Before you buy items that expire shortly, call to find out what days your pantry distributes and if they can handle cold items.

Stock up on staples.

The Osceola, Iowa, Full Gospel Church Pantry opens every Tuesday morning at 8 a.m. "By 9:30, all the bread and milk is gone," says James Sheesley, coordinator, who founded the pantry to honor his mother's dream of helping the poor. These items are nutritional mainstays and disappear quickly from the shelves:

- Milk
- Bread
- Fresh fruits and vegetables

Focus on essentials.

Expensive items or foods with built-in protein are favorites of every food pantry. Prioritize products that can be easily prepared by seniors or children, or that provide a full meal in one can or box.

- Chunky soup with meat
- Stew
- Tuna
- Peanut butter
- Canned pasta with meat
- Cereal
- Oatmeal

Think toiletries.

Remember that pantries distribute more than just food. Low-income families need toiletries and personal care items, too.

- Toilet paper
- Paper towels
- Tissues
- Shampoo*
- Conditioner*
- Lotion*
- Laundry/dish soap
- Diapers
- Toothpaste
- Toothbrushes
- Deodorant

*Bring home unopened, single-use bottles from hotel stays to donate.

Consider the season.

Seasonal items can be great donations, as long as you don't wait until the relevant months are over. In Iowa, cold-weather gear is a great addition to pantries.

- Coats
- Gloves or mittens
- Hats
- Quilts or blankets

Don't shy away.

Exotic or nontraditional items are fine to donate, as long as they don't require lots of other ingredients to make them edible. It's also appropriate to donate dozens of one type of item. Food pantries sometimes put out recipes or prepare ingredients in a plastic bag when they have plenty of one single item.

- Ketchup
- Mustard
- Salad dressing
- Spices
- Nuts

Be safe.

If an item is expired, your food pantry won't distribute it. The same goes for home-prepared food, since it could contain bacteria. "Whenever we get donations, we go through every item to make sure they are still viable to put on the shelf," says Bill Friedow of the Britt Area Food Bank. Also consider the nutritional value of your donations, staying away from empty calories. Most food pantries won't accept these items:

- Expired food
- Dirty or dented cans
- Home-canned fruits, jams or jellies
- Meat frozen by donors
- Home-baked goods
- Junk food

A good rule of thumb: If you wouldn't eat something, don't expect someone else to eat it.

Keep it up.

Food pantries are always in need of donations. And the items they distribute move fast. It's better to donate small bags a few times a month than to give a large gift once or twice a year.

"We are really blessed," says Tina Huinker of the Greater Area Food Pantry at Calmar. "When we need something, it always seems to just show up."

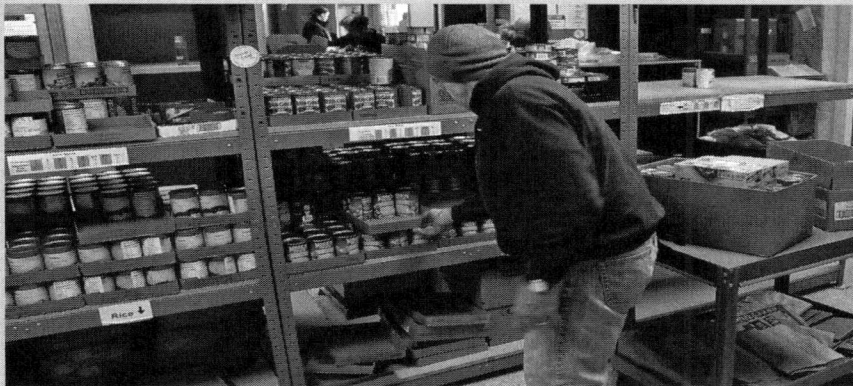

A volunteer helps stock shelves at St. Mary Family Center.

Fresh or Canned?

Both have their place in food pantries—and in low-resource family households. Fresh produce typically is higher in nutrients but has a limited shelf life. Canned foods last longer but often have more sodium and sugar. Here's a quick comparison of some of the most popular vegetables in heartland kitchens.

Green Beans*		Potassium (K)	Vitamin C	Sodium
	Raw	211 mg	12.2 mg	6 mg
	Canned	162 mg	4.1 mg	376 mg

Peas*		Potassium (K)	Vitamin C	Sodium
	Raw	354 mg	58 mg	7 mg
	Canned	263 mg	19.3 mg	459 mg

Sweet corn, yellow*		Potassium (K)	Vitamin A	Sodium
	Raw	292 mg	271 IU	22 mg
	Canned	226 mg	74 IU	305 mg

Tomatoes, orange*		Vitamin C	Sodium	Sugar
	Raw	25.3 mg	66 mg	0 g
	Canned	22.3	307 mg	5.71 g

*One cup

Source: USDA National Nutrient Database for Standard Reference

The Face
of Hunger

SNAP: Myth vs. Reality

While grassroots programs help the hungry, federal aid is essential in alleviating food insecurity. And it may work differently than you think.

Matt Russell is the state food policy project coordinator at the Drake University Agricultural Law Center. He also co-owns and operates Coyote Run Farm with his husband Patrick Standley near Lacona, Iowa. We sat down with him to talk about SNAP, the federal food assistance program.

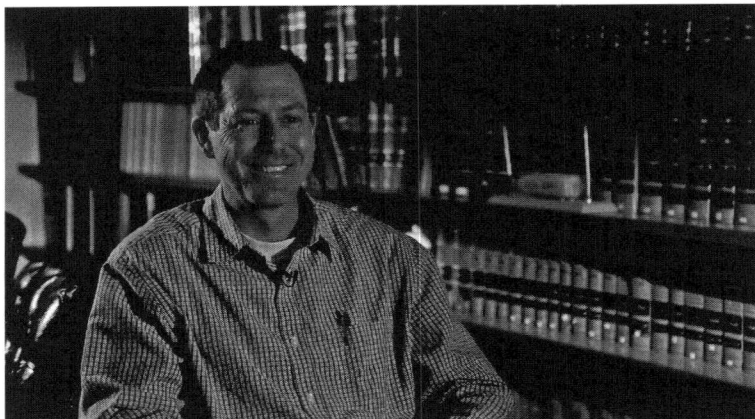

Matt Russell, state food policy project coordinator.

Q. You've been a vocal advocate of the Supplemental Nutrition Assistance Program (SNAP), known elsewhere as food stamps. Why do you feel so strongly about the program?
A. When I was in high school in the 1980s during the farm crisis, my parents' bank failed. That was a stressful time for my family as well as the entire community. One of the things that was very helpful was this: The school superintendent made a strong appeal to members of the community and explained that it was a benefit to the school if families who qualified would sign up for free and reduced-price lunches.

My parents did that, and it made a difference for my family. With three kids, it was a difference of 12 to 15 dollars a week. That was a significant amount of money when there was really not a lot of money in the household. What made it work was that the superintendent said, "This is a benefit to the community."

When people sign up for SNAP and are able to put food on their table, it is a benefit to that family, but it's also an important benefit to the entire community.

Q. In what ways?
A. Instead of going to buy milk and bread and eggs and fresh produce and things that people use SNAP benefits for, those dollars are then freed up to do some other things that that family needs to do.

It could be their heating bill, it could be their car insurance, it could be gas in the car to get to work. The dollars go into that grocery store through SNAP, and it frees up dollars to go into the community.

We're just not doing a very good job of talking about those families and indicating to those families what a benefit it is to the whole community when they use the program in that way.

Q. What misperceptions does the public have about SNAP?

A. I think one of the biggest misperceptions is that it's a government handout, and that in some way people who receive SNAP benefits are doing something wrong. Maybe the stigma is that they're lazy and they should be working but they're not—that this is a free handout.

Q. If that's the myth, what's the reality?

A. The reality is that many of the families on SNAP have a member or more than one member who is working, or they're recently out of work.

The reality is that the families using SNAP have happened to fall on hard times. It could be because of medical reasons—they have a health condition that's causing them to be unemployed, and they're experiencing that whole chaos that is a medical crisis. It could be people who have recently lost their jobs. It could be working moms with

"TAKE A SNAP FAMILY AND A FAMILY NOT USING SNAP, AND CHANCES ARE THEIR BUYING HABITS ARE GOING TO BE VERY SIMILAR."

one or two children, but they're working at minimum-wage jobs that qualify those dependents to have SNAP benefits. That's what those families look like.

They're all around us, and they're contributing members of our community. We need to empower them to use the benefits the best that they can for their family and thank them for using those benefits, because it's a benefit to the community.

Q. That's a very different way of looking at the program. What other misperceptions do you see?

A. Another big misperception about the SNAP program is that families are using those benefits in ways that are much less healthy. Let's just be blunt—that they're buying crap, buying Mountain Dew and pop and candy bars. They're buying unhealthy food

and living an unhealthy lifestyle, and we're supporting that as taxpayers. There are a lot of people out there telling that story, and that's just not true.

For the people using SNAP, the way they use food dollars mirrors the way the rest of the community uses their food dollars. So you take a SNAP family and a family not using SNAP, and chances are their buying habits are going to be very similar.

Now there are a couple of problems. Many people using SNAP live in places where they don't have access to healthy food. Obviously, if you don't have access to fresh produce or you have to drive a long distance to get it, you're probably going to consume less fresh produce. So once you control for the fact that many of these families live in places where access is very difficult, you find that they're

"SEVENTY OR EIGHTY PERCENT—A WIDE MAJORITY OF PEOPLE IN THE U.S.—ARE SUPPORTIVE OF PROVIDING ASSISTANCE AROUND FOOD AND HUNGER. IF...YOU HAVE THAT MUCH ENERGY AND SUPPORT FOR ANTI-HUNGER ISSUES, IT'S A TREMENDOUS ORGANIZING OPPORTUNITY."

using their benefits very similarly to how the rest of the community is buying food. If we empower the community to eat healthier, those SNAP families will follow right along.

Q. How do you empower a change in eating habits?
A. Over the last five years or so, a number of places around the country have done pilot programs where they've taken SNAP benefits and matched them with additional resources. Most of these have been at farmer's markets like Wholesome Wave on the East Coast, which developed a program called double value coupons. A SNAP family could use their benefits to get a dollar's worth of produce, but when they did that, they got two dollars' worth of produce using a voucher coupon.

Data shows that SNAP families will eat healthier and will double up on fruit and vegetable consumption when their SNAP dollars get double the value. What's exciting is that that incentive is now part of the 2014 Farm Bill, institutionalizing this across the country. So we're going to see that happening in a much bigger way.

Q. What is needed to continue alleviating hunger in this country?
A. On a societal level in the U.S., hunger is really about inequality. When you break it down and you control for a lot of different things, the bulk of hunger in the U.S. is about income. What's important about the hunger debate is that 70 or 80 percent—a wide majority of people in the U.S.—are supportive of providing assistance around food and hunger.

They are supportive of using government to do that; they are supportive of using churches and emergency food, and of themselves participating in strategies to help eliminate hunger. If the problem is income inequality and you have that much energy and support for anti-hunger issues, it's a tremendous organizing opportunity.

We're now seeing creative programs, and we're seeing successful government programs. That's the most important thing.

FOR MORE INFORMATION about SNAP, visit **www.fns.usda.gov**.

The Facts About SNAP

Here are a few basics about how the SNAP program works—plus some surprising statistics.

- **SNAP offers benefits** to people who are working for low wages or part-time, or who are unemployed, receiving welfare or other public assistance payments. It also offers benefits to the elderly, disabled, low-income and homeless.

- **The program is administered** through the local offices of state public assistance agencies.

- **Benefits are based on** the U.S. Department of Agriculture's Thrifty Food Plan, which estimates the cost of buying food for healthy, low-cost meals. The estimate changes annually to reflect current food prices.

- **A SNAP household's benefits** depend on the number of people in the household and the amount of monthly income left after certain expenses. SNAP benefits are meant to supplement the amount a family spends on food—not supply the entire amount.

- **SNAP benefits can be used** only for food and for plants and seeds to grow food.

- **Benefits can be used** at farmer's markets. Not all markets are set up to accept SNAP, but this is changing rapidly.

By the numbers...

Average monthly benefit per SNAP household in Iowa in 2009: **$258.11**

Average monthly benefit per SNAP household in Iowa in 2013: **$246.24**

Average monthly benefit per person in Iowa in 2009: **$118.56**

Average monthly benefit per person in Iowa in 2013: **$116.28**

Monthly average number of persons in Iowa participating in SNAP in 2009: **295,106**

Monthly average number of persons in Iowa participating in SNAP in 2013: **420,344**

Percent increase from 2009 to 2013: **42**

Percentage of SNAP households nationally that include a child, or an elderly or disabled person: **76**

Maximum gross household income allowed for SNAP eligibility: **130%** of the federal poverty guidelines

Percentage of SNAP households nationally with gross income at or below 100% of the federal poverty guidelines ($19,530 for a family of three in 2013): **83**

Percent of SNAP households with gross income at or below $14,648 for a family of 3 in 2013: **75%**

Average gross monthly income for SNAP households: **$744**

Length of time an able-bodied, unemployed person without dependents can receive SNAP benefits: **3 months** in any three-year period

Source: www.fns.usda.gov/snap/facts-about-snap

Feed Iowa First

A single mom strives to keep her family fed while working toward food security for all Iowans.

We talked with Sonia Kendrick of Hiawatha, Iowa. Kendrick, the single mom of two young girls, is studying for a master's degree, working on weekends, and building an organization called Feed Iowa First to establish urban donation farms and gardens throughout the Cedar Rapids area. For the time being, she is enrolled in the SNAP program to help her family, even while she's working to feed others in her community.

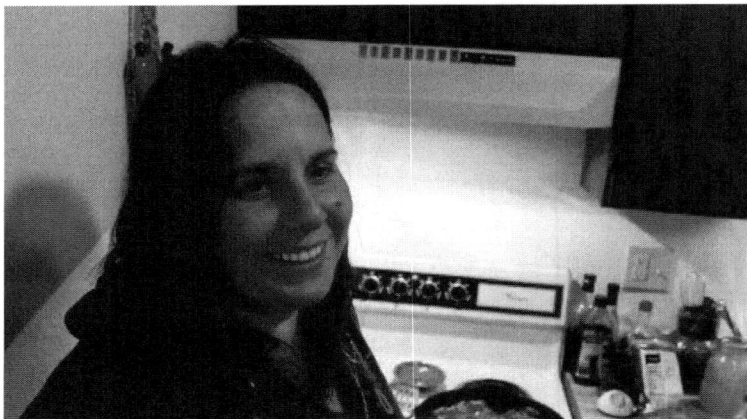

Sonia Kendrick is the founder of Feed Iowa First, which grows food for low-resource people in her community.

Q. What does food insecurity mean for you and your daughters?

A. I haven't always had to access SNAP benefits. It wasn't until I got divorced that I had to go on it. I work weekends for a nonprofit called Discovery Living, where we help mentally and physically disabled adults. It's basically like being a mom. I get paid to sleep there and take care of them. So I can get my 40 hours in during the weekend, then I farm during the week. My girls know I'm busy, but I try to convey to them why.

Q. How does Feed Iowa First work?

A. I started Feed Iowa First when I was in school at Iowa State. What we do is we grow vegetables on underutilized land, and we donate them to food banks, where the food goes out to food pantries.

We are farming all over the city. We are advocating for change in our municipal laws and ordinances regarding farming. The city's been working with us.

In Linn County we have 25,000 people who go to bed hungry. And to feed them the minimum allotted vegetables, we need to farm about 500 acres.

I don't have 500 acres. I live in an apartment. We did a Geographical Information Survey in conjunction with Iowa State University, and we found that there are over 800 acres just surrounding churches in Cedar Rapids, Marion and Hiawatha. So it's not really a problem of land.

Every year I write every seed company you can think of to get donations for the year. So the vegetable seed is free. We use Rockwell Collins land, GE

Capital land, several churches' land, and we just continue to use underutilized land. We rotate throughout the city.

Q. What do you believe is at the root of the hunger issue in this state?
A. Understanding hunger in Iowa is understanding the demographic of the people who are hungry. We're all different, and we have different circumstances.

Food security is national security. If your people are hungry, they're not going to be very restful, and they're not going to be good citizens. In America, hunger is hidden.

If you go to a third-world country, you see people who are rail thin, and you say, "That's hunger." The reality of it is that our food is so calorie-dense and nutrient-deficient that we are starving. People are hungry, and they keep eating. But the food they're eating—there aren't nutrients in it, so they never feel satiated.

We see fat people, and we say,

"IF WE WOULD START LOOKING AT PEOPLE WHO ARE MORBIDLY OBESE AS PEOPLE WHO ARE BASICALLY STARVING TO DEATH, MAYBE WE WOULD CHANGE THINGS."

"Look at that lazy slob. Look at that person who can't control themselves." They don't look at the root of the problem. There may be other emotional problems attached to it. But the likelihood is it has to do with poverty.

If we would start looking at people who are morbidly obese in our communities as people who are basically starving to death, maybe we would change things.

Q. You've served in the military. How did that experience impact your view of hunger?
A. When I was in Afghanistan, I got to see firsthand what hunger

looks like, and what people will do for hunger. We had families there who hadn't eaten in maybe three weeks. They would run across mine fields so they could meet the bread truck. They would eat out of the bottom of Dumpsters and drink out of puddles—not because they didn't know better, but because that's what they had.

So when I come back here, I find out my people are hungry, but in a way that I hadn't imagined.

Q. Do you think the hunger problem can be solved?
A. I actually think the biggest barrier to solving the hunger problem in Iowa and everywhere is the belief that it cannot be solved, so we continue to put Band-Aids on it and stop looking at the root of the problem.

I believe that hunger is an issue that can be solved, and that one day our descendants will look back and see that we were hungry and think, "What a barbaric bunch of people."

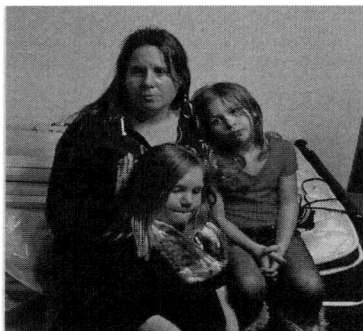
Kendrick and her daughters
Madeline and Danielle.

That is what I would want to see, because I don't think it's necessary to have hunger.

We have so much land, and our land is so much better than anywhere in the world. Nobody should be hungry here, especially when we're standing on gold. We're standing on gold, and we just mow it. Let's change those underutilized spaces into production for our people.

Q. You're growing seedlings in your bedroom to use for Feed Iowa First. How much can you accomplish this way?
A. Even though we live in an apartment and we don't have a lot of money, we can still make a big difference. So here we have 20,000 celery plants, and they'll all be planted for the hungry in our community. If I can do this—and I have Post-Traumatic Stress Disorder—then anyone can really make a difference in our community.

Everything here will go into the food bank. There's already about 4,000 tomato plants started here. It doesn't take a lot of space. It just takes a lot of patience.

Q. Why are you so committed to helping the hungry?
A. I feel like I still have a purpose when I'm helping people in my community. I'm still serving my country, but I'm doing it as a farmer. When I came back from Afghanistan, it was really difficult for me to transition because I have a hard time relating to the idiosyncracies of our modern life. Things like "Dancing with the Stars" aren't even on my radar. When I deal with people who have hunger issues like myself, that's a real need to me. It's worth doing whatever I can.

Q. What do you want to teach your daughters?
A. If you want to do something, you've got to figure out a way to do it.

I want them to be resilient, I want them to be problem solvers, I want them to be not afraid. And capable, very capable.

Feed Iowa First

Sonia Kendrick is thinking about hunger far beyond Iowa's borders. In addition to raising vegetables for the hungry, Feed Iowa First helps beginning farmers get a start. Here are Kendrick's reasons why:

- The global human population recently hit seven billion. The increased competition for fuel and food will only continue to increase the price it takes to import that food.

- Farmers need to increase food production 70% by 2050 in order to feed the projected nine billion people.

- Feed Iowa First provides an opportunity to those who desire to grow our food in the future.

For more information, visit **www.feediowa1st.org**.

Hidden Hunger:
America's Veterans

Tom Sparks never expected to be on food assistance. Or to be a single dad of a ten-year-old daughter. Or to have Post-Traumatic Stress Disorder (PTSD). But more than 20 years after serving in the Gulf War, this former Marine is living the life he never expected, trying to make ends meet with the help of his veteran's disability pay.

Like many people who are food-insecure, Sparks wouldn't fit the profile on paper. He has a degree in horticulture from Kirkwood Community College and lives in an apartment in a pleasant Cedar Rapids, Iowa, neighborhood with his daughter Nellie.

But PTSD—a condition that wasn't recognized, much less treated, when Sparks came home from the war in 1993—has made it close to impossible for him to live a "normal" life. For the first four months after his discharge, he moved back in with his mom but couldn't sleep in the house. "I found myself digging holes and sleeping in them. That was comfortable for me, and I slept with my rifle, too."

In the past 20 years, he's spent time homeless, surviving on what he could hunt, and he's tried twice to commit suicide.

Sparks' situation with food insecurity is not uncommon for veterans. According to 2011 census data, about 900,000 veterans across the U.S.

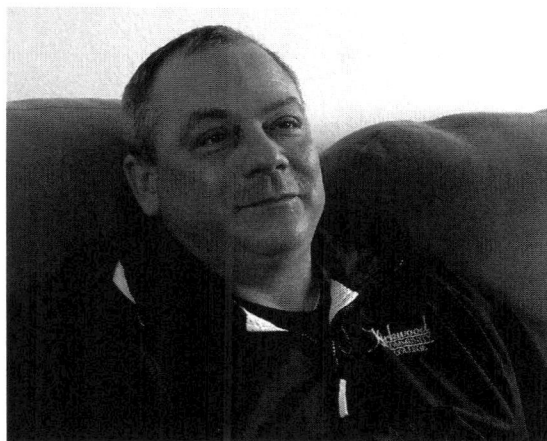

A veteran of the Gulf War, Tom Sparks has struggled with Post-Traumatic Stress Disorder and food insecurity since returning to the U.S.

rely on the Supplemental Nutrition Assistance Program (SNAP). They're just one segment of the population that often is overlooked in discussions about hunger, demonstrating the misconceptions and lack of awareness about what food insecurity in the U.S. really looks like.

The Center on Budget and Policy Priorities finds that households with a veteran who can't work due to a disability are about twice as likely to lack access to adequate food than households without a disabled member.

As with other Americans who qualify for SNAP or utilize emergency feeding programs in their own communities, poverty is at the core of the problem.

"WHEN I WAS HOMELESS, THERE WAS ONE TIME WHEN I LIVED IN THE WOODS, AND I WOULD HUNT OR FISH FOR FOOD. BUT THEN I GOT KIND OF TIRED OF THAT AND CAME BACK INTO SOCIETY A LITTLE BIT. I WAS STILL JUST NOT USED TO IT."

Considered 70 percent disabled by Veterans Affairs due to PTSD, Sparks hasn't been able to hold a job.

"The slightest thing would set me off," he says, "like if the supervisor yelled at me. Instead of dealing with the conflict, I would just leave."

With the help of his doctor, Sparks learned that PTSD has many symptoms. "With me, it's anxiety, sleep disturbance, severe depression, not able to be sociable, unlikely to be productive in a worklike setting," he says.

After five months on the front lines, those symptoms made it hard for Sparks to sleep or associate with people. "Basically I felt like part of me died over in the Gulf War, so I was definitely not the same person at all," he says.

Now that he's a single dad, his views on home-lessness and hunger have changed. He packs his daughter's lunches and relies on assistance from the VA for groceries.

"I don't really care about myself," he says, "but I always think about her first. I have always thought about other people before me.

"Especially being in combat, you always think about your buddy instead of yourself. I'd throw myself on a grenade for my buddy. That's the way I am. That's the way I'm always going to be."

Hunger Among Veterans: By the Numbers

In 2011, percentage of recent veterans who reported service-connected disabilities that affect their ability to provide for their families: **About 25**

Percentage of veterans who served in Iraq and Afghanistan since 2001 who were food-insecure in the past year: **More than 25**

Those reporting very low food security: **12%**

Sources: Center on Budget and Policy Priorities, Cambridge Journals

Helping America's Veterans

You can be part of the solution to help those who have put their lives on the line for our country. Here are a few ways to start.

1. Hire a veteran. Numerous programs provide support to companies that are interested in hiring vets. Check out the following:

• *America's Heroes at Work.* A hiring toolkit helps employers who may be confused or overwhelmed by the process of hiring veterans. Important steps include designing a strategy, creating a welcoming workplace and actively recruiting veterans. **www.dol.gov/vets/ahaw/**

• *The U.S. Department of Labor.* Explore resources for both employers and veterans, including information on employer obligations and veterans' rights. **www.dol.gov/dol/topic/hiring/veterans.htm**

• *Society for Human Resource Management.* SHRM offers assistance to HR professionals looking to find, hire and retain skilled members of the military. **http://shrm.org/hrdisciplines/staffingmanagement/articles/pages/military.aspx**

2. Help veterans "stand down." This term, taken from the battlefield where soldiers "stand down" to rest, refers to events that provide food, shelter, clothes, employment referrals and medical screenings for homeless and unemployed veterans.

Find a Stand Down program—or start a new one—through the National Coalition for Homeless Veterans at **www.nchv.org/index.php/service/stand_down/**.

3. Fight hunger among veterans. Feed Our Vets establishes food pantries across the nation, which distribute free groceries to veterans and their families at regularly scheduled times. Enlist in the Feed Our Vets army and donate money or food, volunteer at a pantry or start a Feed Our Vets Food Pantry program in your community. **www.feedourvets.org/enlist/**

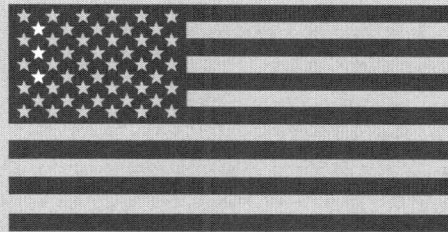

Grocery Shopping 101

How do you eat healthy on a budget? Answers can be found in supermarket aisles—and the lessons are universal.

For Head Start parents in northeast Iowa, grocery shopping now makes a lot more sense, thanks to supermarket tours conducted by members of the Northeast Iowa Food and Fitness Initiative and the Head Start Parent Educator.

According to Haleisa Johnson, early childhood program coordinator with the Initiative, the tours are designed to help parents stretch their food dollars and eat more nutritiously—a combination that some people say is mutually exclusive.

"A lot of people don't know how far fast-food dollars will go to create a fresh meal," Johnson says. "We focus on helping parents eat healthier on a budget, knowing there will be benefits in health and alleviating obesity."

Organized by Johnson and her colleagues, the tours are educational in nature. Not only do participants learn more about foods available, but they receive budget tips, information about reading food labels and ideas for using foods in healthy ways.

The tours are well received in an area of Iowa where the need is acute. Across the U.S., 28.5 percent of Head Start children are overweight or obese. In northeast Iowa, it's 38.9 percent.

"We have to start early and educate the parents," Johnson says. "How many three- to four-year-olds buy groceries and make decisions about meals?"

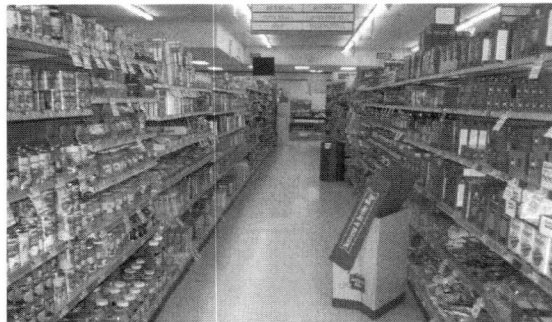

Think you know how to spend a food budget wisely? There's more to grocery shopping than meets the eye.

The problem is compounded by another statistic that is higher than the statewide average: the number of parents working minimum-wage jobs. "Iowa has the highest rate in the nation of parents working outside the home," Johnson says, "and it's even higher in northeast Iowa. Plus, parents are working at minimum-wage jobs—and paying for day care."

In other cases, the parents are young mothers still in high school, or single moms who don't have much support from family and friends. Combine this with society's general lack of education in food science and home economics, and many parents simply don't know how to make smart choices in the grocery aisle.

That's where the tours come in. Follow along with some of the key points from a typical tour, and see what you learn along the way:

Q. Which is the better buy: A bag of apples for 99¢ a pound, or individual apples, also priced at 99¢ a pound?

A. It depends, Johnson says. Will you use a larger quantity? If there's any chance some will go to waste, buying smaller quantities makes more sense. Are you cutting them up in salads or serving them whole as snacks? A bag might have smaller apples, which could mean more individual servings.

Q. When is canned food a good choice?

A. It offers a convenience factor, Johnson says. Plus, it has a long shelf life, and it can offer a better price point (for example, canned pie filling may be cheaper than making your own).

But be sure to read the food labels. Look for differences such as fruit in its own juice or in heavy syrup. If you have high blood pressure or diabetes, avoid canned goods that have added salt or sugar.

Q. Is frozen better than canned?

A. It depends. Compare the price points, and consider whether you have the freezer space. Some frozen foods don't have preservatives, yet they'll last in the freezer for a while. And they give you the option of serving out-of-season fruits and vegetables without paying a premium price.

Q. What are the main considerations in buying dairy?

A. Look for natural vs. added sugars. Strawberry milk, for instance, may sound appealing and healthy, but it's a sweetened drink. Look for added sugar in yogurt, too.

To stretch your budget, check the expiration dates. The store may discount dairy products if they're close to expiring, but they can be frozen and used when you're ready.

Even individual-size containers of yogurt can be frozen and thawed like an ice cream treat.

Q. Are all whole grains created equal?

A. No. The package may say it's 100% whole grain, but look on the ingredient label to be sure.

Q. Should every meal include meat?

A. Meals should include some form of protein, but that can come from eggs, beans, lentils and meats. Consider cutting back on meat by introducing Meatless Monday Meals.

> Check **www.choosemyplate. gov** to see how much protein is recommended for adults and children, along with other nutritional guidelines.

Offering Grocery Store Tours in Your Community

Can the Northeast Iowa supermarket tours be replicated?
Of course, says Haleisa Johnson. She offers these tips for success.

Tap into Head Start or another group of parents.

Promoting tours to the entire community doesn't work, Johnson says. Identify and contact existing groups of parents through churches, library story hours or schools. Then work with the parents' schedules to find the best time for the tour.

Offer an incentive to participate.

Low-resource parents may work more than one job and often are busy with their kids' activities. Give them an extra reason to come to the tour. Johnson offers a $20 gift card (sometimes donated by the grocery store where the tour is held).

Go into the tour with a plan.

Johnson and her volunteers started with the Cooking Matters program (**www.cookingmatters. org**) and adapted it to the needs of their participants.

Provide a challenge.

At the end participants are given a limited time to shop for a meal's worth of food for four that is healthy, represents all the food groups and costs less than $10 total.

Have volunteers on hand to help.

Equip them with calculators to help with figuring costs per pound during the challenge.

Keep the group small.

You don't want to clog grocery aisles—and the group needs to be small enough so that everyone can hear.

Conduct the tour where participants shop.

Find out which grocery store is most commonly used so the tour will be as relevant as possible.

Have a translator on hand if needed.

And take into account the differences in cooking among ethnic groups. Typical Midwestern meals are not the norm for people from other cultures.

Don't be surprised if the group expands during the tour.

Johnson has noticed other people listening in—an indicator of how practical the information is, and how much we all have to learn.

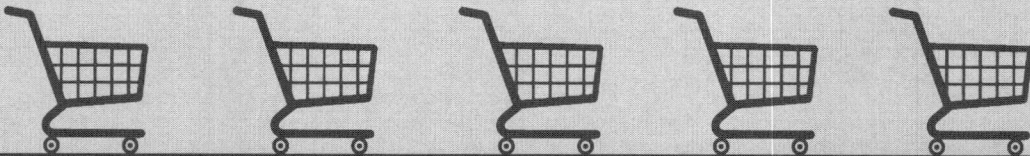

Resources

For more information about the Northeast Iowa Food and Fitness Initiative, including their grocery store tours, visit **www.iowafoodandfitness.org**.

Reaching Out to the Elderly

Volunteers from Pella founded a mobile pantry to reach residents in rural food "deserts" and seniors citizens who can't travel to the city pantry.

In southeastern Marion County, a quartet of tiny rural towns sits some 20 minutes from the nearest grocery store, a half hour from the closest food pantry. Here, where cornfields and county roads stretch for miles, nearly one in five residents are senior citizens; about half are over the age of 45. Industry and other jobs long ago deserted these rural communities, which most residents have called home their entire lives. Farms surround them, but hunger is ever present.

Uncovering that hunger, however, can be a difficult task. Ginny Stralow, a volunteer for the Southern Marion County Mobile Food Pantry, was distributing groceries in Attica when an elderly man told her no one in town was hungry. "Yes," she replied, "but aren't there people who, if they had a little help with their food, could pay their other bills more easily?" The man quickly agreed.

The face of food insecurity in rural Iowa is often just such a senior citizen—someone who has worked hard his entire life but is still struggling to make ends meet near the end of it. "That is the case for a lot of people we are serving," says Stralow, "people who may not be hungry but have to choose between buying food and something else. So the mobile pantry makes it easier for them."

In the U.S., 15 million people over the age of 50 are food-insecure. Nearly 1 in 12 seniors

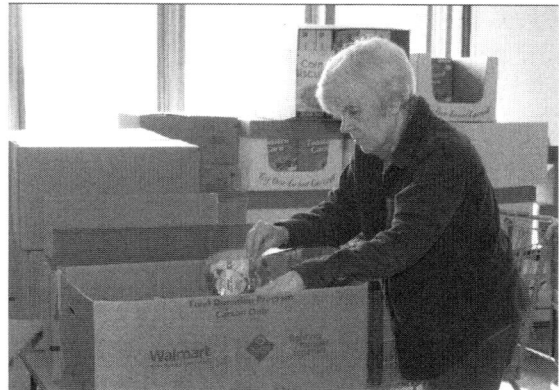

Volunteer Lee Collins packages groceries for the Southern Marion County Mobile Food Pantry distribution project.

Photo: Barbara Ashton

over age 60 are hungry; two-thirds of those live above the poverty line. Many have to choose between buying groceries and paying for expensive medications. According to the Food Research and Action Center, elderly people who are food-insecure are 2.33 times more likely to report fair or poor health. Food insecurity among seniors increases disability, decreases resistance to infection and extends hospital stays.

The Southern Marion County Mobile Food Pantry didn't set out to reach the elderly in their county. At the Second Reformed Church in Pella, a few congregation members got together after a sermon on poverty to brainstorm ideas on how to help the hungry. "Ginny was thinking we should come up with something more than just carrying our bags up to the altar once a month to donate to the Pella Food Shelf," says Jim Zaffiro, a volunteer with the mobile pantry and a professor at Central College.

Second Reformed Church created a hunger task force in the spring of 2014. One of the first ideas was a mobile food pantry to address the great need in the southeastern quarter of the county, where people without the time or transportation couldn't make it to the Pella Food Shelf on Tuesday mornings.

Partnering with Melissa Zula of the Food Shelf, the task force began distributing food in May. Over the summer, the number of volunteers and the number of households receiving food quickly ballooned. And the founders began seeing a trend among the people they were feeding: The majority of them were senior citizens.

"The mobile pantry is not necessarily targeting the elderly, but the net effect is that it's helping the elderly population in these communities," says Zaffiro.

"Older Iowans who are living alone, or who are raising a grandchild, or who may have recently lost their job, are among the most vulnerable Iowans increasingly facing challenges to get enough food and adequate nutrition," says Kent Sovern, state director of AARP Iowa.

The mobile pantry visits Bussey, Hamilton, Attica and Harvey every third Wednesday of the month, when food dollars and SNAP benefits are running low. Located in a rural food

Break Out of the Box

Don't limit yourself to nonperishables such as boxes and cans. Like the task force passing out produce and protein, try incorporating fresh food in your plans to feed senior citizens, some of whom may no longer cook or shop for groceries.

Host a free lunch or dinner. First Lutheran Church in Cedar Rapids has served hot meals on Saturday nights for 25 years.

Deliver door-to-door. Homebound residents appreciate nutritious food delivered warm. Meals on Wheels is a good model that can be replicated on a smaller scale.

Think frozen. Seniors who struggle with cooking may be able to heat up a frozen meal, which can be stored for weeks and brought out when the fridge is empty. The Connections Area Agency on Aging offers a menu of 20 frozen meals for those without a senior center in their area.

Help a neighbor. Do you know any seniors who have trouble feeding themselves on a regular basis? Connect them with one of Iowa's Area Agencies on Aging, which serve community meals and deliver to the homebound, at **www.iowaaging.gov**.

Explore additional ideas. Visit **www.driveto endhunger.com**.

THE FACE OF FOOD INSECURITY IS OFTEN A SENIOR CITIZEN, SOMEONE WHO HAS WORKED HARD THEIR ENTIRE LIFE BUT IS STILL STRUGGLING TO MAKE ENDS MEET NEAR THE END OF IT.

"desert," residents have few grocery options, with convenience stores and gas stations often charging more and offering less. Some seniors don't own cars; others no longer drive or are physically unable to get across town, much less across the county. For these residents, the mobile pantry reaches them right where they most need help: at home.

Starting out, members of the hunger task force connected with citizens in the target towns who could act as community organizers. In Attica, the volunteer fire chief welcomes both pantry volunteers and hungry residents to the fire station during pantry hours. He stows away bags of food to deliver to seniors who can't leave their homes and encourages people who help out neighbors to take extra. "There is a mobile dimension to the mobile pantry, even within the local town," says Zaffiro.

In addition to the typical boxes and cans, the grocery sacks are packed with produce from the gardens of congregation members, as well as high-quality protein. The task force knows that nutritious food is especially important for seniors and older adults, who often face health problems linked to diet. As the mobile pantry continues to grow, the task force is strategizing on how to address "the higher than expected need among the elderly," says Zaffiro.

One of the biggest challenges they face is the justified pride of these senior citizens. Having lived through times of scarcity and worked for everything they own, many do not like the idea of taking something for nothing. "Some of these elderly people will say, 'Give it to somebody who needs it more than I do,' even though they are quite food-insecure and deserving," explains Zaffiro. "You have to be a little more sensitive and proactive in targeting them."

Stralow and the other volunteers try to make the mobile pantry as welcoming and comfortable as possible. They chat with the residents, forging relationships that grow from month to month. They don't want to be seen as the "big city" coming in to solve a problem. Instead, the task force listens to the people they are serving, learning about their lives and their needs. "It's about building community and building ties and building trust, as much as it is about distributing food," says Zaffiro.

Mobilize and Move Out

Consider following the example of Pella's Second Reformed Church. A mobile food pantry can reach rural residents without access to grocery stores or a town pantry.

Connect with local organizations, especially groups already distributing food in your community. A food pantry or service club may want to expand to rural areas. Second Reformed Church partnered with the Pella Food Shelf, which helped supply food with money the task force raised.

Contact community leaders. Find out what the target towns most need, and when and where the food would best be distributed. The hunger task force found site coordinators in each of the four towns. They didn't limit themselves to churches, so that residents of all denominations would feel comfortable stopping by. "We are trying to get past some cultural barriers. A lot of it has been forging those connections, person to person," says Zaffiro.

Find volunteers. The hunger task force inspired huge enthusiasm and support among members of Second Reformed Church. But they also relied on high school students, Boy and Girl Scouts, and members of other churches to help pick up provisions from the Food Bank of Iowa in Des Moines, unload them in Pella and pack them into sacks for delivery. Other community members donated food or money to the cause. Overall, more than 100 people have been involved in the project.

Encourage volunteers to go mobile. Although you may need only two or three people to bring groceries to the town on pantry day, it's important that volunteers see the good they are doing. Stralow urges the people who help unload food and pack the sacks to come along to the towns to meet the residents.

Time your visits right. Find out when the groceries will make the most impact. Often, the need is greatest near the end of the month, when budgets are running low. With recent cuts in the Farm Bill, SNAP benefits aren't stretching as far as they used to for low-income people.

Be committed. Don't create a mobile pantry or any other initiative unless you are in for the long haul. "We aren't going to start, do it for a couple months and then say, 'Sorry, but we're not going to feed you anymore,'" says Stralow. "People are depending on us to help them. And we need to keep doing that."

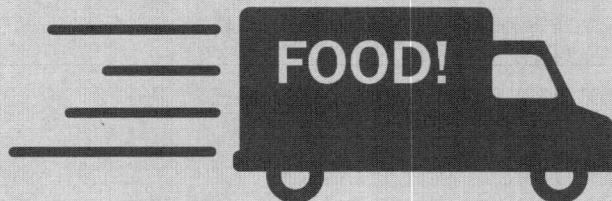

FOOD!

The ABCs of Alleviating Hunger

Learning About Food ASAP

The After School Arts Program includes a culinary component that helps kids find the fun in eating healthy.

Alayna Schutte spent an April afternoon at the grocery store. Whole wheat tortillas were on her shopping list, as were sunflower seeds, olive oil and cheese. But the bulk of the groceries in her shopping cart were vegetables: stalks of fresh broccoli, bright yellow and red bell peppers, asparagus spears, onions and carrots.

Later that afternoon, this member of FoodCorps is taking over the kitchen at St. John's Lutheran Church in downtown Des Moines, along with

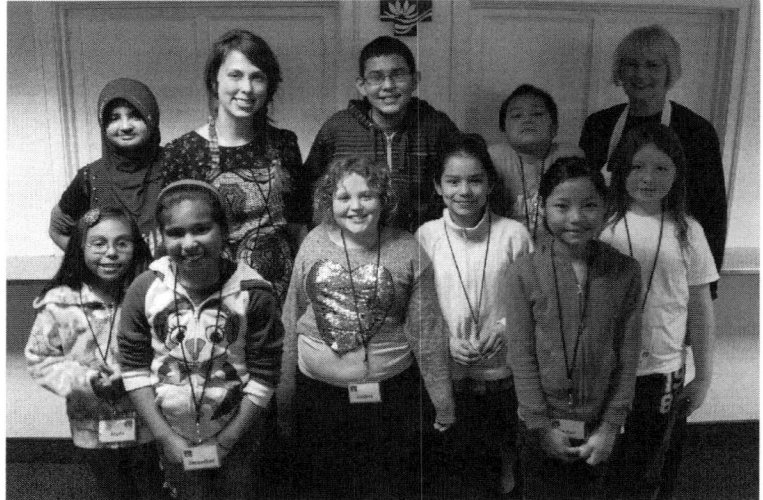

Front row (l to r): Jayda Bernardino, Jacqueline Bernardino, Lindsey Simmons, Genesis Henriquez, Eh Paw, Kaylee Dean. *Back row (l to r):* Nida Afzal, ASAP Teaching Artist and FoodCorps Member Alayna Schutte, Daniel Contreras, Eh Kaw, ASAP volunteer Janet Elwer.

elementary school students involved with the After School Arts Program (ASAP). She's helping them chop up those veggies for kid-friendly quesadillas, and teaching them which part of the plant each vegetable represents.

The students gather around one of the industrial work tables, where the vegetables fill big bowls and colanders.

The children vary in height by at least a foot, attesting to the growth spurts between third and fifth grades. They're about to get a crash course in plant biology—a test that's not for anyone who has been out of school for a decade or two.

Carrots? They're the root, which holds the plant in place and soaks up water. Bell peppers are fruits, which protect the seeds inside. And how about broccoli? The flower.

"What do flowers do?" Alayna asked.

"Look pretty," said one young girl.

"Right," Alayna said enthusiastically. "And the beauty is important because it attracts bees and…"

"Pollinators," says an astute student.

"Right!" Alayna says, clearly impressed with this group's knowledge. It turns out there are six plant parts: roots, stems, leaves, flowers,

THE HOPE IS THAT STUDENTS WILL BE EXPOSED TO NUTRITIOUS EATING HABITS AND TAKE THEM HOME, ALONG WITH HEALTHY RECIPES THEY CAN SHARE WITH THEIR FAMILIES.

fruit, seeds.

And over the next hour, the students would not only learn those parts and what they do, but they'd chop, dice, sauté and bake them all into quesadillas, making friends with vegetables in a way their parents might never have thought possible.

This is one of the aims of ASAP, which attracts more than 700 students from 12 Des Moines schools each academic year to participate in a variety of enrichment classes. Some students might attend sessions on songwriting or comic books. But the kids who get into the culinary class are lucky—it's the most popular program of all.

It's easy to see why, as Alayna and a volunteer direct the students—all decked out in aprons— to use plastic serrated knives to dice and chop the vegetables at stations around the kitchen. There's a quick lesson on safety, then the kids go to work on all those roots, stems, leaves, flowers, fruit and seeds.

A particularly hot onion overwhelms one young lady. "Give your eyes a break, and wipe your eyes with your apron," Alayna advises.

Over the chatter and chopping, Alayna invites a couple of students to start sautéing. And when the dicing is done, half the class vies for position at the sink to wash the knives and cutting boards. Again, this is something parents may not have seen before.

"Never put a knife in soapy water," Alayna reminds the students, who are endlessly polite and seem remarkably savvy about kitchen protocol.

Students are chosen for ASAP for a number of reasons, says Executive Director Michelle Bolton King. "They may have a budding talent, a special interest, or there may be a perceived need. These are students who may be struggling in other aspects of their lives," she says.

While not all are from food-insecure homes, some of the children do deal with hunger issues, which makes the culinary class doubly meaningful.

The hope, says King, is that students will be exposed to nutritious eating habits and take them home, along with healthy recipes they can share with their families.

All that chopping and plant-part identification

ALL THAT CHOPPING AND PLANT-PART IDENTIFICATION CAN GIVE THE KIDS A VESTED INTEREST THAT MAY SPILL OVER WHEN THEY GO GROCERY SHOPPING WITH THEIR PARENTS.

can give the kids a vested interest that may spill over when they go grocery shopping with their parents and request a head of broccoli or a bag of spinach. In any case, it gives them a healthy snack, since the class—as always—concludes with sampling the food they've just helped prepare.

Alayna directs them to load their tortillas with as many veggies as possible. "I want all the plant parts in my quesadilla," she says. "The more veggies, the more cool points you get."

And now, pulling the finished products from the oven, it's time to try them—an experiment that goes considerably better than most parents might have predicted.

By the end of the afternoon, the kids have eaten their plant parts, done a cheer to fix those parts in their minds and headed home with a muesli snack kit to share more healthy food with their families. All in all, not a bad couple of hours' work to increase nutrition education and alleviate hunger.

FOR MORE INFORMATION
Who could replicate the ASAP culinary arts class? Schools, churches and youth organizations. For additional information, visit **www.asap-dsm.org**. And to learn more about FoodCorps members, visit **www.foodcorps.org**.

Plant Parts Cheer!

How do you help kids remember the parts of a plant (or learn them yourself)? Practice this Plant Parts Cheer, acting out each part along the way.

Start the cheer slowly, then repeat it three times, speeding up each time.

"We've got our roots!"
(Stomp your feet.)

"We've got our stems!"
(Move your knees together, Charleston style.)

"We've got our leaves!"
(Flutter your arms at your sides.)

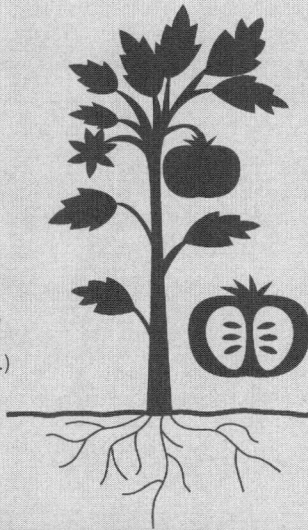

"We've got our flowers!"
(Wave your arms gently above your head.)

"We've got our fruits!"
(Curve your arms at your sides.)

"We've got our seeds!"
(Wiggle your fingers with your arms to your sides.)

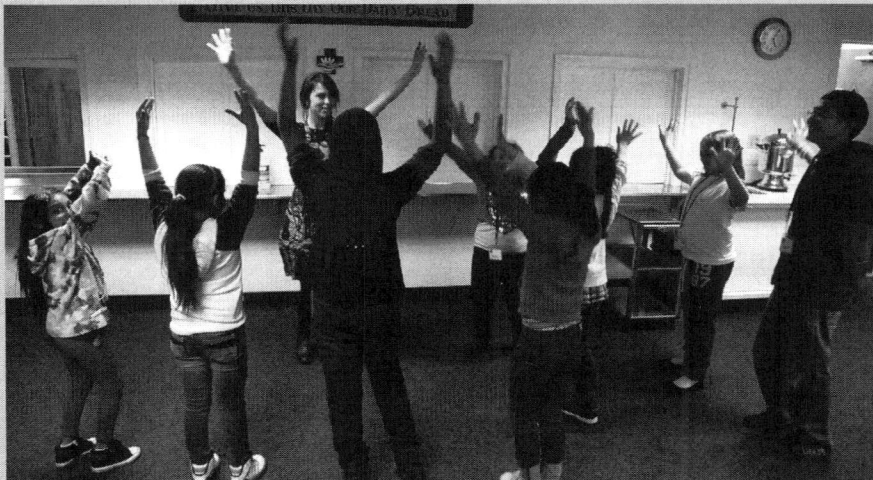

Alayna Schutte and her ASAP students act out "We've got our flowers!" as part of the Plant Parts Cheer.

Plant Parts Quesadillas

From the ASAP Culinary Arts Program

Makes 12 quesadillas
12 whole wheat 6-inch tortillas
1 medium onion, diced
1 bunch of asparagus, diced
1 lb. of carrots, chopped
2 heads of broccoli, chopped
1 10-oz. bag of fresh spinach
2 bell peppers
   (orange or red, if available), chopped
4 roma tomatoes, chopped
2 8-oz. bags shredded mozzarella cheese
Salt and pepper to taste
Extra virgin olive oil
Sunflower nuts

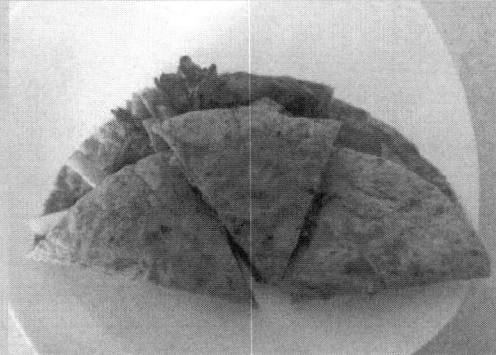

Photo: The Naked Food Life

1. Preheat oven to 350 degrees; lay tortillas out on baking sheet.

2. Sauté diced onion in 1 tablespoon of olive oil until translucent.

3. Add diced asparagus, carrots, broccoli, salt and pepper, and sauté 5 to 10 minutes longer.

4. Remove from heat; place sautéed vegetables into tortillas.

5. Top with spinach, bell peppers, roma tomatoes, sunflower nuts and shredded cheese.

6. Fold or roll tortilla to close quesadilla.

7. Bake in the oven for 5 to 8 minutes or until cheese is melted.

Good to Know

The After School Arts Program culinary class is held at St. John's Lutheran Church in downtown Des Moines in part because the church has a large kitchen. The program, though, could be taken on the road, and portable stoves could be used to make it mobile.

3 Ways to Get Kids to Eat Healthy Foods

Chelsea Krist, FoodCorps member at Hillis Elementary School in Des Moines, shares what she's learned about getting kids excited about foods they've never tried before. *Hint: No trickery required.*

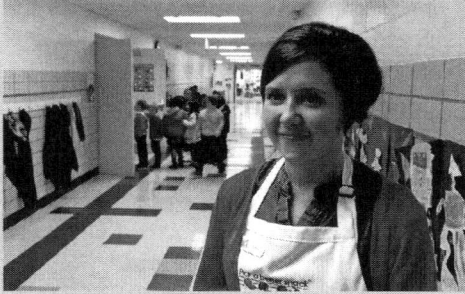

Chelsea Krist is known as the "snack lady" at Hillis Elementary.

Keep it simple. "Just make it a commonplace thing," Krist says. Something as easy as letting kids wash and chop carrots gives them ownership of the process. "It takes away the scare factor."

Connect foods to children's books. For instance, Krist read *The Cat in the Hat* with a group of third-graders, then made kabobs to look like the classic Seuss character. "We alternated bananas and strawberries on a skewer, then added a tiny crimson apple for the head, toothpicks for whiskers and raisins for eyes." Want more ideas? Krist recommends Pinterest, where you'll find other book-inspired snacks.

Mix it up. Think of new ways to introduce healthy ingredients into foods kids love. Krist's students harvested squash, tomatoes, kale, broccoli and carrots from the school garden, loaded them onto whole wheat tortillas, added a little cheese and baked them for hearty and healthy veggie quesadillas. "They couldn't get enough of them," she says.

Think kids won't eat kale?

Think again. Chelsea's fifth-graders not only tended kale in the school garden, they made posters about this super food—then wrote and performed a rap song about it at a school assembly.

"A room of kids chanting 'K-A-L-E' is, indeed, a rare and remarkable sight," Krist says. Here's a recipe that was a big hit with the kids.

Kale Chocolate Chip Cookies

1 firmly packed cup of torn kale leaves
2 1/2 cups whole wheat flour
1 cup old-fashioned oats
4 tsp. baking powder
1/2 tsp. salt
2 cups brown sugar
1 cup (2 sticks) unsalted butter, soft
4 eggs
2 T. vanilla extract
2 cups dark chocolate chips
1 cup walnut halves (optional)

1. Preheat oven to 350 degrees.
2. In a food processor, pulse kale 10-20 times until finely chopped. Set aside.
3. In a bowl, combine flour, oats, baking powder and salt. Set aside.
4. In a large bowl, beat butter and sugar with an electric mixer, on a low speed, until thoroughly combined. Continue running mixer on low, and add eggs one by one until just incorporated. Add vanilla extract.
5. Combine butter/sugar/egg mixture with dry ingredients. Add kale and half the chocolate chips. Mix all together until just incorporated.
6. Using spoon, drop dough onto greased baking sheet 2" apart. Distribute remaining chocolate chips onto each cookie and, if using walnuts, place walnut half on top of each cookie.
7. Bake for 12-15 minutes or until cookies are firm around the edges but still slightly soft in the middle.
8. Cool and enjoy! *Makes about 40 cookies.*

From the Farm to the School

Nearly 200,000 kids in Iowa qualify for free or reduced-price meals through the National School Lunch Program. That's 40 percent of the total kindergarten through 12th-grade population.

For many of these students, school breakfast and lunch are the only times they get reliable, healthy meals.

The Farm to School Program of the Iowa Department of Agriculture and Land Stewardship (IDALS) strives to provide students with nutritious, fresh food—especially fruits and vegetables—straight from local farmers. Their success is especially important for the children who rely on school lunch as their primary source of nutrition.

The Farm to School program gives children from all backgrounds access to nutritious food, while at the same time benefiting local farmers. In Iowa, 460 schools participate in the program. There are 27 chapters established in the state. Approved Farm to School chapters can apply for up to $4,000 in initial funding from the state.

"It's a win-win for students, growers and the Iowa community," says Tammy Stotts, Farm

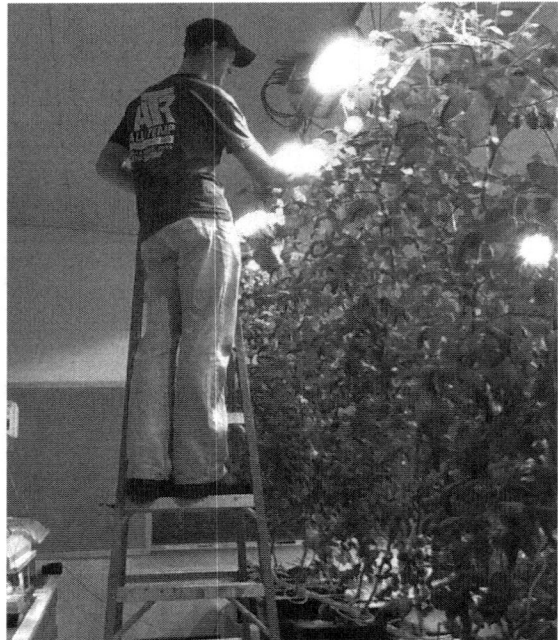

Photo: Mike Elwick, Old School Produce Company

Food now grows where students once did. In a former school building in Vinton, the Old School Produce Company uses a hydroponic system to grow tomatoes (pictured), lettuce and other veggies for salad bars in the Vinton-Shellsburg School District year-round.

to School coordinator with IDALS.

The need for fresh, local produce is especially important today, when less than 30 percent of Iowa children eat the recommended five

ACCORDING TO EXISTING FARM TO SCHOOL PROGRAMS, FRESH FRUITS AND VEGETABLES RANK AMONG STUDENTS' FAVORITE MEAL OPTIONS.

or more servings of fruits and vegetables daily.

Over the past 30 years in Iowa, the percentage of overweight children has tripled. Low-income kids are especially at risk. One national study found that children from lower income households were more than twice as likely to be obese than children from higher-income households.

Establishing good eating habits early in life is essential for these children. "Many students may not get the opportunity at home to try different kinds of fresh, locally grown produce. Without this opportunity, they will not likely seek it as adults," says Stotts.

But according to existing Farm to School programs, fresh fruits and vegetables rank among students' favorite meal options.

Some programs include school gardens, nutrition lessons and farm visits for students. The Farm to School program also helps fund initiatives promoting Iowa-grown apples and FFA chapters that found school gardens.

The school district in Independence, Iowa, has been committed to Farm to School for seven years. The campus has had a garden where students help grow and harvest fruits and vegetables, and it's building a new greenhouse with a hydroponic system, allowing them to grow produce into the winter.

Jessica Weber, food service director for the

Did You Know?

- Only about a fourth of Iowa children consume the recommended five or more daily servings of fruits and vegetables. School lunches are an excellent way to introduce more fresh produce in their diets.

- Local foods supplied by farmers may include eggs, cucumbers, lettuce, tomatoes, strawberries, melons, cheese, dairy and ground beef.

- When a Farm to School program is introduced, participation rates in the National School Lunch Program typically increase.

- Students who eat Farm to School meals waste less food than students who eat other hot lunches.

- Farm to School programs offer educational benefits, such as farm tours, visits with local farmers and recycling programs. They also can help children better understand the impact of food on their lifelong well-being.

"IT'S AMAZING THAT EVEN IN A SMALL RURAL TOWN LIKE VINTON, KIDS DON'T NECESSARILY KNOW WHERE THEIR PRODUCE COMES FROM."

district, is in charge of getting bids from local farmers for tomatoes, yogurt, strawberries and more.

Weber credits community support for the program's success in Independence. A local farmer donated $13,000 to build the greenhouse. Volunteers come in over the summer to cut and freeze strawberries for the school year. That dedication pays off when children pick out their lunch. "They love knowing that it's local. They are so much more likely to eat it that way," says Weber.

In an old abandoned schoolyard in Vinton, Iowa, retiree Mike Elwick started a small vegetable farm called Old School Produce Company. Because of the connection, Elwick invited local schools to take tours of the farm. That led to visits from food service directors and then to sales of his produce for school lunches.

Elwick put in a hydroponic system in an old classroom to grow lettuce, cherry tomatoes, peppers and cucumbers for the salad bar over the winter.

Elwick is encouraging other farmers in the area to consider selling to schools, too. He organized a meeting over the summer between producers and food service directors in Benton County to facilitate the partnership.

"It's amazing that even in a small rural town like Vinton, kids don't necessarily know where their produce comes from," he says. "Here in Iowa, we are the breadbasket of the world. Why aren't we growing the produce for our kids here?"

FOR MORE INFORMATION
If your school wants to work with local farmers, or if you're a farmer who would like to supply food to schools, contact the Farm to School Program at the Iowa Department of Agriculture and Land Stewardship at **515/281-5783**, or at **www.IowaAgriculture.gov.**

Driving Away Hunger: Teens Take Charge

Every November, hundreds of teenagers come together to scream and cheer. They aren't rooting for a football team or shouting for a favorite band. Instead, they hoot and holler as a giant banner is unrolled—reading, last year, "521,115 pounds."

That was the total amount of food they had collected over the previous six weeks for the hungry in their community.

The Student Hunger Drive was founded in 1986, when Pete Puhlmann of Davenport, Iowa, president of Lujack's Autoplaza, took a breather from the car sales business. Thanksgiving was coming up, and food was on his mind—but not just the traditional turkey dinner.

Instead, he was thinking about the people who would go without enough food that holiday season. He decided to get a few local high schools involved in collecting cans.

Today, the Student Hunger Drive regularly brings in more than 500,000 pounds of food in the Quad Cities (QC)—a metro area spanning both banks of the Mississippi River in Illinois and Iowa. In 2013, 18 high schools in the region participated.

"The Student Hunger Drive is a project that teaches students leadership and community service while fulfilling a community need—feeding the hungry," says Denise Hester, executive director of Student Hunger Drive, Inc. All the

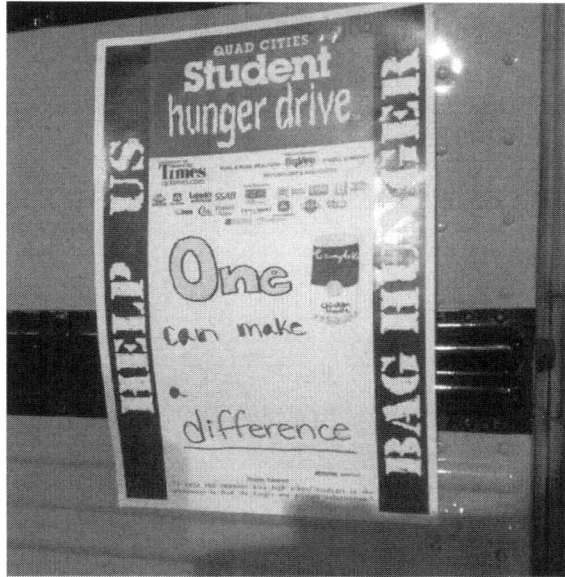

The Student Hunger Drive teaches Quad City high school students about hunger in their hometowns. In 2013, teens collected more than 500,000 pounds of food for the hungry in their communities.

food collected through the drive is donated to the River Bend Foodbank, which serves 22 counties in Illinois and Iowa.

The drive behind the Drive is the high school students, who throw themselves into the project each year. Schools compete against one another in categories based on enrollment, and the schools are eager to win the crown in their division. That involves planning events to promote the Drive, purchasing food with monetary donations, organizing and packing the items and, finally, delivering the provisions to the Foodbank.

Each school has at least one faculty advisor and several student leaders. To raise money, they plan dances, soup and chili dinners and even, in the case of one imaginative school, a male beauty pageant.

Learning to Drive

Over nearly 30 years, each succeeding generation of QC high school students has taken on the challenge of easing hunger in the Midwest. Matt Clark of Des Moines graduated from a QC-area high school in 2005.

"Participating in the Drive every year left my classmates and me with a sense of accomplishment," he says, "because we saw the direct results of our efforts: People in our local community received the food we collected. It had a clear impact on their well-being."

First- and second-place schools in each division win cash prizes, as does the school earning Most Improved.

All high schools that raise more than three pounds per student are awarded $500 to help them recoup the costs of the Drive—such as renting a semitruck to haul the food—or to donate to another charity of their choice.

In 2013, Bettendorf High School took first place in Division A, with 41.5 pounds per student—a total of more than 60,000 pounds of food. "I enjoy rallying the students around the cause and getting our entire school on board," says Katie Hansen, biology teacher and student council advisor at BHS.

A Community Hunger Profile

The River Bend Foodbank has distributed 25 million pounds of food since 1982. A recent study of its clients reveals startling facts about food insecurity.

40% of households have at least one full-time employed adult

39% are children younger than 18

10% are children age 5 and younger

46% report choosing between buying food and paying utilities

40% report having to choose between food and medical care

78% are below the federal poverty level

13% are homeless

10,000 people receive food assistance in any given week

"THE SCHOOLS THAT HAVE THE GREATEST SUCCESS ARE THE ONES THAT REALLY UNDERSTAND THE ISSUE OF HUNGER— UNDERSTAND THAT THEY HAVE FRIENDS OR NEIGHBORS OR FELLOW STUDENTS WHO ARE HUNGRY."

A Mighty Hunger

Thanks to the annual Student Hunger Drive, the Quad Cities is more conscious of its hungry inhabitants than many Midwestern towns. Still, lack of awareness about food insecurity is common.

Hester lives in Bettendorf and finds silence on the subject during the rest of the year. "I think hunger is one of those issues that is not talked about very much," she says.

Since she became executive director of the Student Hunger Drive five years ago, the River Bend Foodbank has more than doubled the amount of food it distributes to over 8 million pounds annually— a huge increase during the recession years, especially as the price of food rose steadily.

Hansen believes that, at the beginning of the Drive each fall, many of her students don't truly understand the needs of their neighbors. The last few years, Bettendorf High School has joined the mobile pantry effort, with students literally handing food to the hungry in their city. "It has been a great experience to actually see and serve the families that receive our donations," says Hansen. "It became more real to me after serving at this event."

Hester says that knowledge is an essential part of the Student Hunger Drive. "The schools that have the greatest amount of success are the ones that really understand the issue of hunger—understand that they have friends or neighbors or fellow students who are hungry," she says.

"Once we get the message out to the schools and get the kids engaged, they just buy in wholeheartedly. They are more than willing to give back."

The students learn to take ownership by watching the rest of their community get involved, including parents, faculty, staff and local businesses.

Alumni keep memories of the Student Hunger Drive alive as they enter adulthood. Hester says she often meets young professionals who say they want to find opportunities to give back the way they did as high school students.

Recalling his days as a student, Clark says that

the Student Hunger Drive took the abstract idea of hunger and made it real. "It helped many of us realize that it's not only people in other parts of the world who wonder where their next meal will come from; it's sometimes our neighbors who have to think about that question."

Spreading the Word

Since 1986, the Student Hunger Drive has spread to other metros around the country—Charlotte, North Carolina; South Bend, Indiana; and Lincoln, Nebraska.

One reason for the Drive's expansion is the experience students get with teamwork, leadership, problem solving and communication. They often work closely with community members and business professionals as they strive to raise money and food.

Hester counsels potential supporters to contact their area food bank to make sure they are not duplicating services. The point of the Student Hunger Drive is to assist the food bank, not take on its responsibilities.

The Student Hunger Drive is funded by local individuals and corporate sponsors. Finding community support is key to starting a Drive in a new city.

Hester says that the Quad Cities knows to look for the Student Hunger Drive every fall, which empowers students on their quest to make a difference in their hometown.

"It's so rewarding to know that you are filling a drastic need in the community," says Hester. "Hunger continues to grow in the Quad Cities, and I'm helping to teach kids to give back."

FOR MORE INFORMATION or to replicate the School Hunger Drive in your community, contact Denise Hester at **563-359-9389** or visit **www. studenthungerdrive.org**.

The Corporate Challenge

Each fall, area businesses sponsor the Quad Cities Student Hunger Drive and provide donations to local high schools. Still, some businesses felt they could do more. As a result, the Student Hunger Drive created the Corporate Challenge to promote community engagement and friendly competition among Quad Cities workplaces.

The Corporate Challenge takes place over four weeks in February, just as the food collected during the Student Hunger Drive is running low.

In 2014, 33 businesses competed in the Corporate Challenge, sponsored by the real estate firm Ryan Companies US, Inc., which provides the funding to facilitate the Challenge.

The businesses—both for- and not-for-profit—conduct internal food drives and raise money from employees. Some have asked staff to pay to dress in jeans for a day or play in a company golf outing.

The John Deere Foundation matched all the donations, leading to a total of more than 150,000 pounds in 2014. Cash donations were earmarked for the BackPack Program, which provides weekend meals for elementary school students (see page 15).

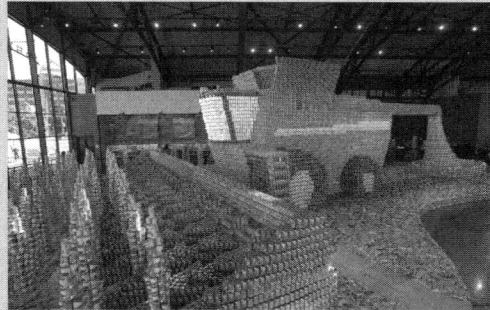

Photo: courtesy of John Deere

In 2012, John Deere won the Guinness World Record for the largest sculpture ever made from canned food—creating a full-size S-Series Combine with 170 tons of cans eventually donated to the River Bend Foodbank. Displayed at the John Deere Pavilion in Moline, Illinois, the structure contained enough cans to feed 450 low-income people for a whole year.

Denise Hester, executive director of the Student Hunger Drive, is happy to see adults emulating the high school students. With the Corporate Challenge, the Drive has spread awareness of hunger in the Quad Cities to another important group of people. "The business community really steps up," she says.

Farming for the Community

Across the heartland, the rural economy has long depended on small family farms. Now, while large farming operations play their role in feeding the hungry, smaller farms are experiencing a resurgence, thanks to Community-Supported Agriculture (CSA).

The basic model is an agreement between a farm and a group of consumers. Each CSA member pays a flat fee up front for a share of the agricultural products grown on the farm, which can include vegetables and fruits, meat, eggs, dairy and bread. Many of these operations farm less than 20 acres of land; some farm only five.

According to the Leopold Center for Sustainable Agriculture at Iowa State University, the average CSA provides enough food for a household of two to four people. The first CSAs in Iowa began in the mid-1990s, and today there are 81 in Iowa, serving an estimated 4,000 households throughout the state.

"CSAs have a very important role in the growth of small-scale agriculture and the expansion of local food systems," says Savanna Lyons, graduate assistant at the Leopold Center. For farmers, a CSA guarantees a certain level of income each season and provides capital early in the spring when the need for seeds and equipment is greatest.

In exchange for the weekly fresh food, CSA members take on some of the risk farmers

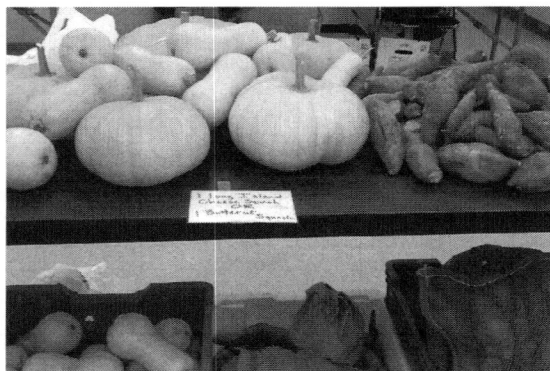

Farm to Folk, a CSA in Ames, Iowa, donates leftover produce to a local food pantry.

experience on a daily basis. If the crop is beset by drought or disease, they may not receive as much or any of what they expected. But the reward is fresh food grown for taste and nutrition, reduced shopping time, knowledge of how their food is grown and a close relationship with local farmers.

CSA members can pay anywhere from $150 to $800 for a share of the farm's produce. Vegetables like tomatoes, peppers, beans and sweet corn are the most common, but members may also receive unusual produce such as kohlrabi or edible flowers. Thus, consumers get a chance to try food they may have passed over in the store.

"Iowa has a ready consumer base of people interested in buying local food, especially in its cities," says Lyons. " Although land and equipment can be prohibitively expensive for grain

MANY CSAS AND OTHER ORGANIZATIONS LIKE FOOD CO-OPS MAKE SURE THEY'RE INVOLVING LOW-INCOME FAMILIES IN THE PROCESS.

farming, CSAs allow farmers to go another route.

"By producing vegetables or other high-value farm products for local markets, new farmers can make a living on a small piece of land and with fewer capital investments," she says.

In Iowa, farmers and their partners have come up with many different ways to involve the community in agriculture. That community encompasses more than paying shareholders. Many CSAs and other organizations like food co-ops make sure they're involving low-income families in the process. Here are three examples of different ways to serve the hungry through community agriculture.

Mustard Seed Community Farm

Inspired by the Catholic Worker movement and Gandhi's teachings, the Mustard Seed Community Farm in Ames is based on a set of values—foremost among them service to the poor.

"We are imagining a world that we wished we lived in and saying: 'Let's just see what happens if we try to live in that world,'" says Alice McGary, a founder and leader of the farm.

McGary and her team grow typical Iowa produce, as well as some unusual fare, on 10½ acres,

some of which is devoted to prairie. They sell a third of what they grow through their CSA, give a third to volunteer workers and donate a third to local food pantries, soup kitchens and shelters. "At the fundamental level, we believe that everybody deserves really good food," says McGary.

As a CSA, it is helpful for Mustard Seed to know what their budget is before the season begins and to be freed from the stress of constant marketing. All three parts of their distribution are important, but the giving of food is more vital to their mission and serves an unmet need in their community. "It is more important for us to be giving food away than selling food," she says.

The proof of that is the 2010 growing season,

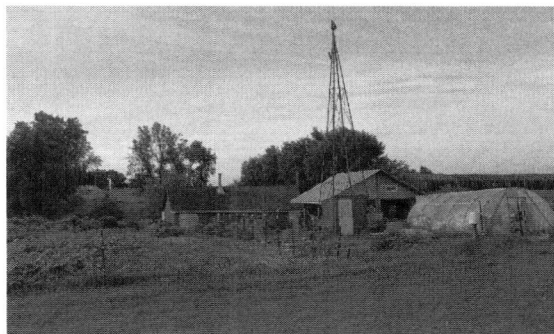

Photo: Kaitlyn Rusca

Mustard Seed Farm

which was exceptionally rainy. Like many farms, Mustard Seed was faced with smaller harvests and produce rotting in the fields. As a result, they weren't giving away as much food to the poor. McGary and her team went to paying customers and explained the situation, offering to refund their money. Instead, the members decided they wanted less food so that more could go to pantries and shelters.

McGary says paying customers have other options. They could still get fresh produce if Mustard Seed didn't exist. McGary notes that some Iowans face food insecurity and lack access to most foods. Even more, she says, "are having trouble buying really good food in Iowa." Vegetables are expensive, require cooking knowledge and need refrigeration, which can be barriers to entry for people who can otherwise afford to feed themselves.

It's easy to get overwhelmed by the problem of hunger in Iowa, comments McGary. The important thing is to do what you can, no matter how small. "Sharing a meal with somebody is a big deal," she says. "Growing and sharing vegetables with somebody because you care about them is a big deal. Maybe it's not going to save the world from hunger, but it might mean a lot to someone."

Iowa Food Cooperative

Born out of the belief that the state needed a better way of getting food to people, the Iowa Food Cooperative began as an online food distribution system in 2008. It offers more than 1,000 products—vegetables, milk, eggs, baked goods, honey, cheese, milk—from farmers around the state in two-week cycles. Members log on to choose the products they want during each cycle. Instead of paying a flat fee up front, the consumers pay for what they order, plus a 15 percent fee that goes toward running the co-op.

The Iowa Food Co-op now has more than 900 members, including 150 producers, the majority from central Iowa. Last year, they sold $250,000 worth of local food to Iowans. Gary Huber, general manager, calls it "food you would like to feed your children" and "food that can dazzle." Some of the producers are certified organic; most are chemical-free.

"We don't say how farmers should farm," says Huber. "All we do is ask them how they are doing what they are doing so that we can make informed choices."

As a cooperative, one of the principles they follow is concern for community. "We are figuring out how we can lead healthy lives as a community," says Huber. "That means all segments of the community, including low-income."

Members of the Iowa Food Co-op can purchase a product online—a $5.75 donation to families in need. Some members do it every single cycle. The money goes into the co-op's budget to cover the fees for low-income members, who purchase using SNAP benefits.

The Supplemental Nutrition Assistance Program (SNAP)—formerly known as food stamps—allows low-income individuals to use their federal benefits to purchase food. CSAs across the state are starting to accept SNAP, and the Iowa Food Co-op has been taking it since the beginning. Nearly 10 percent of their members purchase food using SNAP. Per federal regulations, however, SNAP can only be used to purchase food and cannot cover the fees associated with CSAs or co-ops. The member donations cover those fees, allowing low-income families to use the online service to buy quality, local food.

"We are trying to figure out how to we can use the power of our pocketbooks to change the world to the kind of place we want to live in," says Huber.

Farm to Folk

One of the oldest CSAs in Iowa, Farm to Folk was founded in Ames in 1996 as Magic Beanstalk CSA—a collaboration among five different farmers. Ten years later, it changed its name and its model and became Farm to Folk, which offers CSA shares from three separate farms, as well as a weekly á la carte menu from dozens of other producers.

Farm to Folk sells vegetables, fruits, herbs, dairy and meats that have been produced using sustainable methods. They also strive to educate the surrounding community about nutrition and agriculture.

That devotion to community also manifests itself in the low-income assistance fund, which allows any of the 300 members to donate to low-income families. Those donations go toward a discount on a CSA share or a matching fund for money spent in the á la carte system.

"It's our belief that finances shouldn't be a barrier to getting healthy food," says Marilyn Andersen, coordinator of Farm to Folk. "We want to accommodate people who couldn't afford the full price of the CSA share while still supporting farmers for their work."

Farm to Folk also donates leftover produce—whatever members don't pick up—to the local food pantry. Andersen brings in at least one big box of vegetables a week. Members are enthusiastic about the donation of leftovers, and they let Andersen know when they will be out of town or won't need their entire weekly share. That leaves even more nutritious food for the pantry.

"Getting fresh, healthy food is a good way to stay healthy, and low-income people need that as much as anyone else," says Andersen. "We need to make them feel part of the community, too."

Before You Join a CSA

Put some thought into your food and into these considerations from Savanna Lyons of the Leopold Center.

Prep time. Using fresh produce often means cooking from scratch, which is a rare phenomenon these days. "Making time for this might involve a conscious commitment and some adjustments," says Lyons. On the plus side, these from-scratch meals will cost less and provide more nutrition.

Share size. Depending on your family, you may want anything from multiple shares to part of one. Most CSAs offer a full share that feeds 3-4 people and a half share suitable for 1-2. If you are unsure about how much you'll use, start with the smallest size.

Vegetable storage. You can't just throw produce in the fridge when you get home. You first need to learn to store different fruits and vegetables properly. Some produce—such as tomatoes, sweet potatoes and butternut squash—are best stored at room temperature.

Cooking knowledge. Using unusual fruits, vegetables, honey or cheeses can be tough without recipes and preparation know-how. "If you aren't used to cooking with fresh produce, a CSA can be a good motivation to learn," says Lyons. But don't overwhelm yourself. Consider a cooking class; Lyons suggests finding one through your local ISU Extension and Outreach office.

Excess food. If you don't use all the produce from your CSA share, or if you're going to be out of town, make plans for the extra food. Consider giving your share to a needy neighbor or your local food pantry. Call ahead to make sure they accept produce and to find out what days they distribute.

To find a CSA near you, visit **www.leopold. iastate.edu/csa** and click on "Get the most current directory."

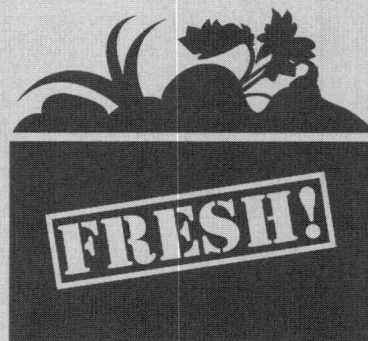

Rescuing Food and Land

Table to Table

Ever looked at all the restaurant food that goes to the Dumpster and wondered how it could reach the people who need it? Table to Table has found the answer.

We talked with Bob Andrlik, executive director of the Table to Table food rescue program in Iowa City, Iowa, about the genesis of his organization, its surprising impact, and what other parts of the country are doing to reduce food waste.

Q. How does Table to Table operate?

A. The organization began in April 1996. There was a group of individuals that had seen something, I believe on CNN, about food rescues and the concept of keeping food from going to waste and what communities can do about it.

That first year, using their own vehicles, they rescued about 40,000 pounds of food—basically bread, bakery, things being recycled off the shelves. That's your access kind of products that you're able to get ahold of when you don't have refrigeration.

From there it just grew, creating the network of donors and the network of recipient agencies.

Now we have about 30 regular donor organizations, including grocery stores, warehouses, hospitals, institutions like schools and universities, and restaurants like Olive Garden, Red Lobster, Panera, Starbucks and Caribou Coffee.

Then what we do is we have about 34 agencies in our circuit of places that we take food to.

Q. What impact does Table to Table make?

A. In 2013, we rescued over 1.13 million pounds of food. That's the raw poundage. Every 1.2 pounds is considered an equivalent meal, so we extrapolate that that's over 941,600 equivalent meals. From that, we're able to come up with the monetary impact to the community. Because we deliver to agencies, not individuals, that's about a $2.56 million impact in terms of dollars saved to budgets. Those savings are passed through to the individuals that come to the agencies. That doubles the impact to about $5.12 million.

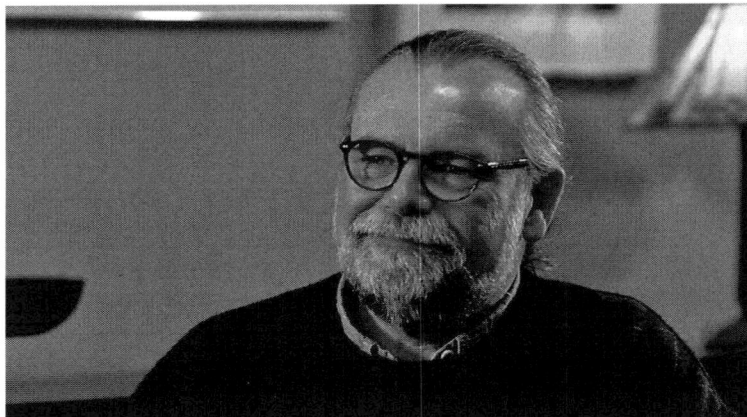
Bob Andrlik, executive director of Table to Table.

"WE'VE RESCUED OVER 12 MILLION POUNDS OF FOOD. THAT'S A HUGE NUMBER. BUT AT THE END OF THE DAY, WHAT I LIKE FOCUSING ON IS THAT WE'RE GETTING FOOD TO ONE PERSON OR ONE FAMILY THAT MIGHT OTHERWISE NOT HAVE HAD IT."

It's a tremendous resource flowing through the community. If we can keep that food from going to waste, it makes a big impact on the lives of people using the food, as well as the agencies striving to provide them services.

That's the kind of volume we're tapping into with a population of 130,000 people. If you have a larger city, it's going to be ramped up per the population and the stores they have. If it's a smaller city, there's less available.

We're also looking at all the energy it took to produce that food, to process it, package it, market it, get it to stores and then, when it's still wholesome and edible, to bury it. It makes no sense when so many people are in need.

Over 100 billion pounds of food in the U.S. go to waste every year. Author Jonathan Bloom of *American Wasteland* has created a snapshot of what that looks like. It's like filling the Rose Bowl from the football field to the top-tier seats every day with food. That's how much is being wasted at different levels for different reasons. Maybe it goes bad due to processing. Or it goes bad before it goes to market. We're focused on the post-marketing aspect.

Q. How important is food rescue in the continuum of food assistance?

A. With food rescue you're taking something that doesn't have any more marketable value. Yet you're leveraging the value back up by distributing it to agencies to support the social safety-net services they're providing. You're also getting it to people who require it to survive. It's a relatively high-impact process without necessarily costing a lot of money.

We're a nonprofit entity and don't charge any fees. We're trying to find funding to cover our expenses from United Way grants and foundation support, and direct and individual donations. That's how we're able to do the work we do. Every dollar that comes in has a $28 impact as it goes out to the agencies and to the individuals and families they're serving.

Q. Are there other food rescue programs like Table to Table?

Eliminating Food Waste at Home

Food waste in the United States is estimated at 30 to 40 percent of the food supply. Some of this food could be going to hungry people rather than filling up landfills and creating greenhouse gases. According to the Iowa Food Waste Reduction Project (iwrc. org/services/food-waste), almost 14% of all municipally landfilled waste is food waste, making it the number one most prevalent disposed material.

What can individuals do? Here's a list of easy ways to reduce food waste at home. For more information, visit the food waste reduction website at www.usda.gov/oce/foodwaste/resources/consumers.htm.

1. Shop your refrigerator first! Cook or eat what you already have at home before buying more.

2. Plan your menu before you go shopping and buy only those things on your menu.

3. Buy only what you realistically need and will use. Buying in bulk only saves money if you are able to use the food before it spoils.

4. Nutritious, safe and untouched food can be donated to food banks to help those in need.

5. At restaurants, order only what you can finish by asking about portion sizes, and be aware of side dishes included with entrées. Take home the leftovers, and keep them for your next meal.

6. Compost food scraps rather than throwing them away.

7. Don't automatically throw out food that has been in the freezer longer than "recommended." Food

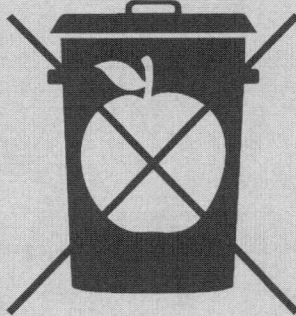

poisoning bacteria does not grow in the freezer, so no matter how long a food is frozen, it is safe to eat.

Foods that have been in the freezer for months may be dry, or may not taste as good, but they will be safe to eat.

So if you find a package of ground beef that has been in the freezer more than a few months, don't throw it out. Use it to make chili or tacos. The seasonings and additional ingredients can make up for loss of flavor.

8. Likewise, canned goods will last for years, as long as the can itself is in good condition (no rust, dents or swelling). Packaged foods (cereal, pasta, cookies) will be safe past the 'best by' date, although they may eventually become stale or develop an off flavor. If food appears moldy or discolored, do not eat it.

— Iowa State University Extension and Outreach, Human Sciences

"OVER 100 BILLION POUNDS OF FOOD IN THE U.S. GO TO WASTE EVERY YEAR. IT'S LIKE FILLING THE ROSE BOWL FROM THE FOOTBALL FIELD TO THE TOP-TIER SEATS EVERY DAY WITH FOOD."

A. There are so many different types and forms of food rescues. In some places, like Seattle, it's part of the solid waste diversion program, so it's part of the municipal structure.

Some large food reservoirs have food rescue as part of their component instead of being freestanding rescues like Table to Table. So there are a lot of different wrinkles to the food rescue process.

For us, it works out well because we have a high percentage of volunteerism in our area of Iowa. We have about 130 volunteers and 67 route slots every week. But the logistics get really complex.

The concept of keeping food from going to waste is really simple, but not every donor donates every day, and not every agency receives every day. You have to factor that in.

What are the times the donors are willing to donate? What are recipient agencies' times to receive it? They have to plan for the rest of the day, so we need to get to them as early as possible so they'll know what to buy if we're not able to provide everything they need.

Q. Why is food rescue important to you?
A. Since 1996, we've rescued over 12 million pounds of food. That's a huge number. But at the end of the day, what I like focusing on is that we're getting food to one person or one family that might otherwise not have had it. There's a whole series of "ones" that add up to the meals provided by the agencies.

Q. Why is now the time to become involved?
A. If not now, when? We know the need is there and the need is growing. We know that wages have been stagnant for so long. We know that we've weathered a terrible recession.

But there's a wonderful resource out there that we can take advantage of just by people taking action. As long as there's a need and the ability to address that need, there's no reason why we shouldn't.

FOR MORE INFORMATION, visit **www.table2table.org**.

How to Create a Food Rescue Program

Food rescue programs are possible thanks to the Bill Emerson Good Samaritan Food Donation Act, which protects individuals and businesses from liability when they donate to nonprofit organizations that feed the hungry.

To start a program in your community, consider the following tips.

- **Talk to others in your community.** What individuals and organizations are already working on food distribution and alleviating food insecurity? This research may lead to productive partnerships and will prevent you from duplicating efforts.

- **Set up a board of directors.** The board can help develop and carry out the mission of your program, as well as helping with fundraising and logistical details.

- **Apply for 501(c)3 status.** As a nonprofit, you can give grocery stores, restaurants and other donors your tax-deductible number, encouraging donations.

- **Contact potential food donors.** This includes grocery stores, convenience stores, warehouses, restaurants, coffee shops—any businesses that may have food to donate.

- **Set up a food collection system.** Recruit volunteers who can go to the donor businesses at the same day and time each week. According to David Wellendorf, volunteer coordinator for Table to Table, it's essential that volunteers be on time, consistent and trustworthy, as they will represent your program and may have unsupervised access to food supplies at the donor businesses. Have volunteers wear name tags with your program's name or logo so employees at donor businesses will recognize them easily.

- **Seek out recipient agencies.** Look for agencies such as shelters and food pantries that can make direct use of the food you collect. Find out what kinds of food they need, and when it should be delivered. For example, if they prepare a large congregate evening meal, they may need the food by late morning so they can begin cooking and know how far the donated food will go.

- **Line up transportation.** To start out, you may need to use your own vehicles (outfitted with coolers for perishable foods). As your program grows, financial donations may help cover the cost of a van or truck.

- **Train volunteers.** Develop a standard set of instructions to simplify the process of bringing new, qualified volunteers on board. Establish a scheduling system that allows you to easily track when volunteers will be picking up and delivering food.

- **Engage in meaningful outreach.** Talk to community members about supporting the program through financial donations. In addition, send frequent communications to local media to spotlight your work and the difference it makes.

- **Expect the unexpected.** Put backup plans in place to deal with weather issues, volunteers who need to cancel at the last minute, transportation problems, and other changes that may effect your volunteer force and scheduling. Being dependable and consistent with donor and recipient agencies is key.

Plant Your Parking

One of the best places to help feed people in your neighborhood may be in your own front yard.

Greg Schmidt has plans for Clear Lake, Iowa. Sure, the community may be known for the Surf Ballroom, the last place Buddy Holly played before his fateful plane crash. Yes, it may be the spot where boaters and water skiers kick back during summer months. And, certainly, it may be the sister community to Mason City, adored by fans of "The Music Man" as River City, Iowa.

But if Schmidt has his way, it will soon have another identity: the national headquarters for Plant Your Parking, a movement encouraging gardeners to plant fruits and vegetables in the parking strip between their sidewalk and the street curb.

The idea just makes sense, Schmidt says. And he's got a whole list of reasons to back him up.

"Most backyards sit under too much tree shade, have storage sheds, clotheslines, patios, lawn furniture, fire pits/grilling areas, flower beds, garages, doghouses/pet areas or other obstructions," he says. In contrast, parking strips often get full sun—the ideal condition for vegetable gardens.

Communities with parking-strip gardens inspire tourism, a tip he picked up from his mom, whose gardens in Garner, Iowa, are so admired they attract bus tours.

Parking-strip gardens offer a great alternative to community gardens because there's easy water

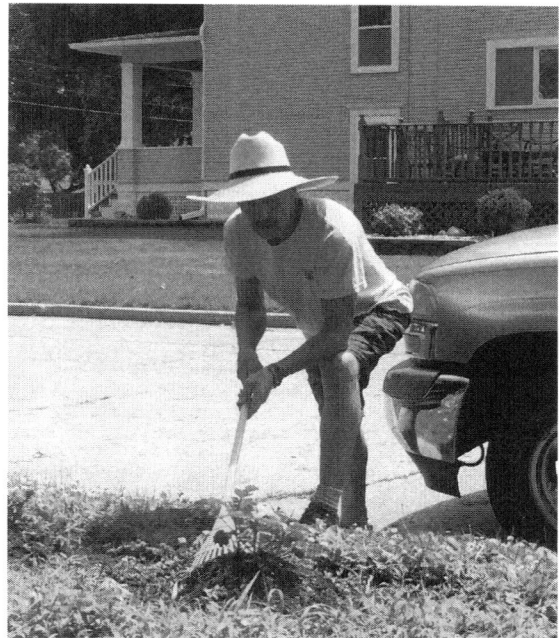

Greg Schmidt prepares the soil for his parking-strip garden.

access—a feature many community gardens lack.

The gardens can cut down on the amount of mowing you need to do, which saves on noise and air pollution.

And planting vegetables out front makes it easy for anyone to pick them, which is the whole point, Schmidt says.

"It's free food for neighbors who walk by and know they can take the produce home." What doesn't get picked by passing pedestrians in Schmidt's front yard goes to local schools and

PARKING-STRIP GARDENS OFFER A GREAT ALTERNATIVE TO COMMUNITY GARDENS BECAUSE THERE'S EASY WATER ACCESS—A FEATURE MANY COMMUNITY GARDENS LACK.

food pantries.

Schmidt, who organizes both film and herb festivals across the state, tried the idea for the first time three years ago, to not-so-great results. "I planted corn and got a citation from the city to cut it down because it blocked the view of oncoming traffic," he says. Since then, he's gotten more savvy about his plantings, and the idea is catching on.

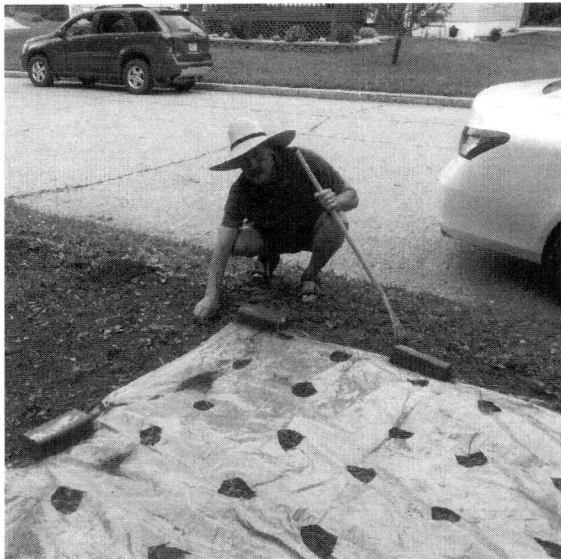

Greg highly recommends weed barrier to prevent one of a gardener's biggest frustrations.

Several of his neighbors have started their own parking-strip gardens, with seeds supplied by Schmidt. And while he hasn't had trouble dispensing raspberries, he finds he has to talk people into picking rutabagas.

Clear Lake is not the only place with parking strips-turned-gardens. The same idea has been proposed in Seattle and Orlando. But Schmidt is leading the local charge toward streets lined with lettuce—and his vision is as big as that corn the city objected to.

"Let's turn Iowa into the produce capital of the world," he says. "If healthy food is cheaper food, it changes things."

And it can all start in your own front yard.

FOR MORE INFORMATION, contact Greg Schmidt via **gregfest@netins.net**.

How Do You Start?

To introduce a Plant Your Parking program in your neighborhood, follow Schmidt's tips:

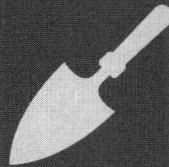

1. Check the rules and regulations in your community. Call the mayor's office to find out what you can and can't do. For instance, most communities prevent planting on street corners, as it impairs visibility for drivers at intersections.

2. Plant low-growing plants like root vegetables to make sure you're not obscuring visibility in any way.

3. Leave a strip of grass between the vegetable bed and the curb. This prevents mud from washing into the street, allows people to stop their cars and get out onto grass and gives city workers access in case they need to dig for utility work.

4. Find a volunteer with a rototiller to prepare the initial garden bed. (Some utilities may come in from the street. Check for buried cables before rototilling.) If you have a large area to clear, contact a local nursery. They may be willing to cut the sod for free if they can take it and sell it.

5. Use weed barrier to keep weeding to a minimum. This will make your life easier and will eliminate the number one cause of discouragement in gardening.

6. Plant bedding plants rather than sowing seeds directly in the ground. They'll grow healthier, and you'll be miles ahead. *(For tips on seed selections, see page 97.)*

7. Border the garden with marigolds. They'll defend against pests and beautify the less glamorous vegetables. Rutabagas, for instance, may be packed with nutritional benefits, but "they are not attractive," Schmidt says.

8. Encourage passersby to harvest the fruits of your labor. This can take a little time, Schmidt says, as people aren't used to helping themselves in other people's gardens. Put up a sign that says "Free Food: Please Pick," and leave plastic bags and berry baskets where people can see them.

9. Enlist volunteer help. Find your own local labor force, such as church members or Boy Scouts.

10. Turn your neighborhood gardens into a destination. Work together with neighbors to name or number your gardens, and identify them with common signage. Set up a tour during harvest season to get publicity and encourage people to pick your produce.

Alleviating Hunger, One Deer at a Time

When the meat first began to show up, no one knew what to do with it. The food pantry coordinators were just as stumped as the patrons. But soon deer meat became one of the most popular items at pantries across the state. Tina Huinker, coordinator of the Greater Area Food Pantry at Calmar, Iowa, has seen hungry Iowans recognize venison for the tasty source of protein that it is. "Now we always run out of deer meat," she says.

The venison comes from Iowa's Help Us Stop Hunger (HUSH) program, which is run by the Department of Natural Resources (DNR). The program serves two worthy objectives: managing the deer population while providing high-quality red meat to needy Iowans. The venison comes from hunters who choose to donate their kills through HUSH.

"The HUSH program is a great wildlife management technique with a tremendous social impact," says Jim Coffey, coordinator of the HUSH program at the DNR. "We are allowing hunters to take an extra deer, and we are managing the Iowa deer population. At the same time, we are directly benefiting needy Iowans."

HUSH began when deer numbers escalated during the mid-1990s. At that time, says Coffey, the population was getting beyond what is called "social-carrying capacity," meaning

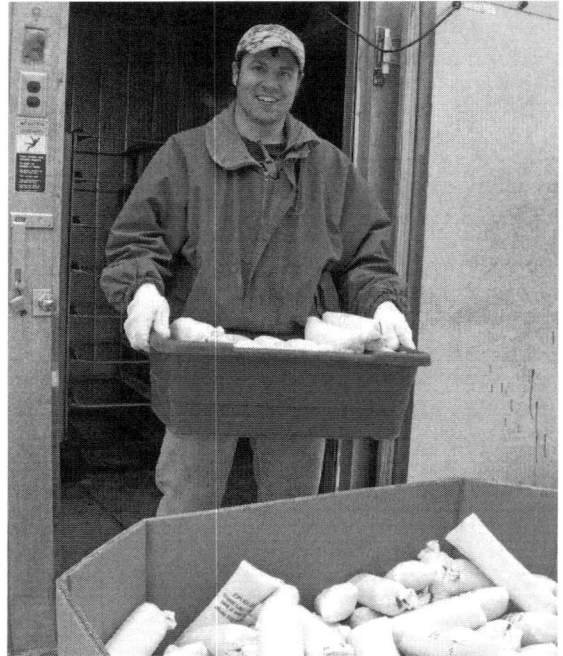

Donated deer are processed by participating meat lockers into two-pound packages of venison. In 2013, the HUSH program supplied 160,000 pounds of meat to pantries.

there were too many deer for humans to tolerate—too many in cornfields, too many in backyard gardens, too many putting drivers in danger on the roads.

When more hunting was suggested, even the hunters were uncomfortable with the idea. "Traditionally, with hunting, people are very ethical," says Coffey. "They don't kill for sport or recreation. They typically kill for purpose,

SOME HUNTERS NOW HARVEST DEER EXCLUSIVELY FOR THE PROGRAM. "THEY ENJOY THE FACT THAT THEY CAN GO OUT AND SHOOT A DEER AND THAT DEER WILL HAVE A PURPOSE...TO HELP SOMEBODY IN THE COMMUNITY."

and that purpose is eating the animals." Killing more than they could eat went against their code.

Donating excess deer to food pantries was a win-win situation. Hunters could purchase additional tags, which allowed them to continue hunting. They could then choose to donate the extra deer if they wished. They are not obligated to donate any meat when they purchase an extra tag. They may also donate the first deer they harvest.

HUSH began in 2003, and since then, 56,000 deer have provided protein for low-income Iowans.

Coffey says the program has been an absolute success for everyone involved. HUSH is a four-way partnership among the DNR; the Department of Agriculture, which inspects the lockers; local meat lockers, which process it; and the Food Bank of Iowa, which distributes it.

Hunters, too, are pleased with the results. Some hunters now harvest deer exclusively for the program. "They enjoy the fact that they can go out and shoot another deer and that deer will have a purpose," says Coffey. "It will go to a

neighbor, to help somebody in the community."

In 2013, hunters donated 4,000 deer through HUSH—about 160,000 pounds of meat. As in Calmar, the venison disappears off pantry shelves almost as soon as it arrives. "The Food

Hunting in the Heartland

To donate deer through the HUSH program, here's what you need to know before you head out.

- Buy a deer permit beforehand, and make sure to hunt in season.
- You can donate any legally taken deer of either sex.
- You must label the deer with the provided tag before you transport it to the locker.
- You may donate only a whole deer, which must be field-dressed and preferably mud-free.
- Once at the locker, fill out a HUSH donation card. There is no charge for the meat processing.

Bank absolutely loves it," says Coffey. "It's one of the greatest forms of protein they get in their system."

The number of donated deer peaked in 2007, when hunters brought in almost 8,500. Since then, totals have been dropping as the deer population shrinks. Coffey is glad to see the gradual decline, since that's what the DNR was trying to achieve. Still, it means less meat for hungry Iowans. Those numbers could rise, however, if more hunters donated what they kill.

A. Jay Winter, education specialist at Springbrook State Park, is an avid hunter and loves to go out in nature with his two sons. "I enjoy the outdoors, the relaxing atmosphere, the bounty of the harvest, the camaraderie," he says. Winter donates one or two deer a season, and he encourages other hunters to donate what they

Buffalo Feast

Deer hunters aren't the only ones who donate their kills to the needy. Since 2003, the Iowa chapter of Safari Club International has harvested bison meat for the hungry through the Jack Hagens Great Buffalo Giveaway (named after a deceased member who helped pioneer the project).

The club wanted to create a humanitarian program by combining wild game hunting with helping the homeless. Each year, the club sells a bison hunt at a South Dakota ranch to an enthusiastic club member.

Other members travel to the neighboring state to help butcher the animal and harvest the other two bison donated by the ranch. All total, that comes to between 1,500 and 2,000 pounds of meat.

"The best part is that it doesn't cost anybody anything," says member A. Jay Winter of Dallas Center. The ranch donates the animals, members harvest the meat and the club auctions off the bison skull and hide to pay for the program.

After the bison is processed at the Frederika Locker, the Safari Club donates the meat—enough for about 6,000 meals—to shelters in Des Moines run by Hope Ministries, Central Iowa Shelter and Services, and Freedom for Youth Ministries.

Every year, Winter takes his wife and two sons down to Bethel Mission to help serve the meat the day before Thanksgiving.

"It really opens my eyes and my sons' eyes that not everybody lives exactly like we do," he says. "Some people are not as fortunate as we are."

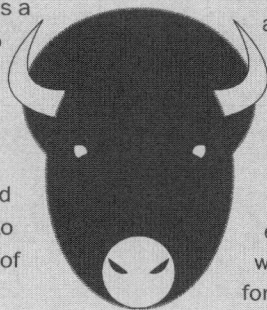

don't eat. He believes the HUSH program is a good use of a natural, renewable resource that helps the hungry and balances out the environment.

"The program keeps alive the tradition of hunting for purpose," says Coffey. "When I shoot a deer, I have respect for that animal—for the circle of life. We are shepherds of this herd."

Winter says donating deer meat is something he would do no matter what, but the HUSH program allows it to occur on a much larger scale, providing a lot more protein for pantries.

After a hunter has killed a deer, he or she takes it to the nearest participating meat locker, which has signed an agreement to work with the DNR. The hunter fills out a donation card, and the locker skins, bones and grinds the meat into two-pound packages of venison for the local food pantry to pick up.

The locker is paid $75 for each deer by the Food Bank of Iowa, which is then reimbursed by the DNR, along with a $5 administration fee.

Iowa is unique among states with similar programs in that it charges all hunters a one-dollar fee when purchasing a deer license. The hunters are accepting of the extra fee, says Coffey, which funds the HUSH program.

Other states require hunters to pay the meat locker themselves or rely on unpredictable donations. Coffey is often asked to advise other states on starting a similar program, and he says Iowa's success is due to its stable funding system, as well as the efficient inspection process and trusted food bank network.

The food pantries receiving venison from the 85 participating meat lockers across the state are all grateful for the infusion of a vital nutrient. Huinker shares ideas for cooking the protein with patrons at the Calmar pantry.

One volunteer brought in lemon-pepper seasoning to cut the gaminess. Barbecue sauce is another favorite. No matter how it's used, Huinker wants the venison to keep on coming from Iowa hunters.

"Please shoot some deer," she says. "We use it. We need it."

FOR MORE INFORMATION, visit **www.iowadnr.gov**.

The Great Pork Giveaway

An Iowa foundation donates protein to people and pantries, giving back to a state that has helped make its hog-farming business a success.

Protein is one of the most difficult nutrients for the hungry to acquire. Meat, especially, is expensive and difficult to store. That fact is distressing in a state that raises nearly one-third of the nation's hogs. Iowa's largest pork producer, Iowa Select Farms, decided to do something about it.

Iowa Select Farms has 550 farms and nearly 1,000 employees across the state. The company's founders, Deb and Jeff Hansen of Iowa Falls, created a foundation in 2006 to help address hunger in the communities where they operate.

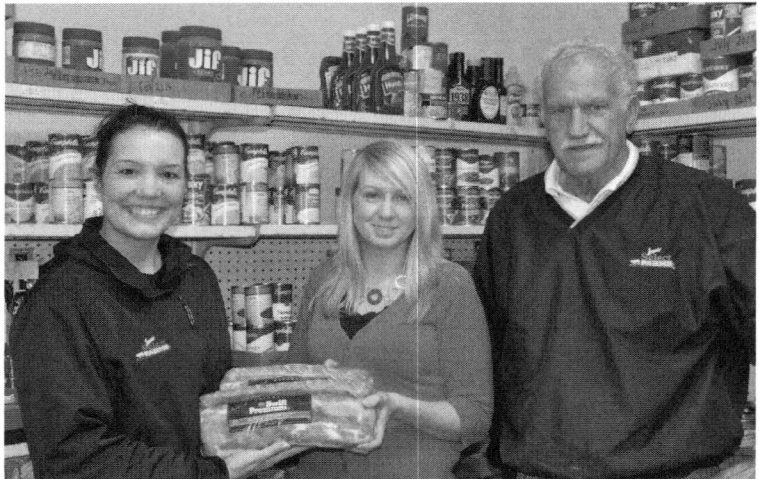

The Emmett County Food Pantry, represented by Program Assistant Jessica Breuklander *(center)*, was one of 50 organizations to receive pork loins from the Deb and Jeff Hansen Foundation last year. The pork loins are delivered by employees of the foundation and Iowa Select Farms, including Jen Sorenson *(left)* and Gary Kramer *(right)*.

"It's a natural fit for us," says Jen Sorenson, communications director for Iowa Select Farms. "As a pork producer here in the state of Iowa, hunger relief is something we can contribute back to Iowans, and especially to the communities where we have farms and people."

This year, the Deb and Jeff Hansen Foundation will donate more than 100,000 pounds of pork to nearly 50 food pantries and other organizations around the state. They provide cases of boneless pork loins—each enough to feed a family several times over. Pork loins are nutrient-rich and recognized by the USDA as a lean protein.

The foundation formed relationships with food pantries across the state, and they distribute as many cases as each pantry needs. Company employees also deliver pork loins into the hands of people who help others, such as nurses who serve the homebound.

"It's hard to put into words the gratitude and appreciation for the pork loins," says Sorenson.

"I know the pantries really enjoy being stocked up and having their freezers full."

In addition to its twice-yearly deliveries—once before the holidays and once in spring or summer when pantries are low—the Deb and Jeff Hansen Foundation issues $5 coupons for sliced ham to elementary schoolkids in the BackPack Program *(see page 15)*. Finally, as a holiday act of kindness, the foundation distributes pork loins at the Iowa State Fairgrounds in Des Moines, in partnership with WHO Radio's "Van and Bonnie Show."

The giveaway begins at 5 a.m. on a cold December morning, and citizens begin lining up in their cars at 2 a.m. In drive-through lines, the foundation hands out a pork loin to anyone who needs one—or who can pass it on to someone else in need. "People take that request very seriously," says Sorenson.

On a comment card sent back to the company, one recipient expressed the gratitude common to the season. "When Santa handed me the pork loin, I just started to cry. It is so wonderful to know there are people who care."

FOR MORE INFORMATION about the Deb and Jeff Hansen Foundation, visit **www.iowaselect.com/ foundation/foundation.aspx**.

Donating Meat

Sharing the gift of protein can be tough. Regular donors should consider canned meats, peanut butter and beans, as they are shelf-stable for months. Monetary donations also allow food banks and pantries to purchase the necessary meat on their own. But livestock farmers can make a difference, as long as they follow regulations.

- **All meat must be processed and inspected.** The pork loins from the Deb and Jeff Hansen Foundation come prepackaged from JBS in Marshalltown. Call your local food bank to find out what you need to do to satisfy their requirements.

- **Learn what the community needs.** Fifty pounds of meat can be enough for a small pantry. "Some of our best efforts are delivering one case of 12 pork loins to a food pantry because that is exactly what they need," says Sorenson.

- **Remember that no gift is too small.** "Don't ever think that because you are a small farmer, you can't make an impact," says Sorenson. "You absolutely can."

Set Free

An unlikely partnership between the Food Bank of Iowa and the Newton Correctional Facility yields thousands of pounds of produce—and a fresh lease on life.

Filling garden beds sometimes requires strange bedfellows—as does filling the stomachs of Iowa's most needy citizens. To accomplish both, Newton Correctional Facility (NCF) and the Food Bank of Iowa have formed a novel partnership.

Three years ago, John Baldwin, director of the Iowa Department of Corrections, and Carey Miller, executive director of the Food Bank of Iowa, discovered that their respective missions actually meshed. The Food Bank of Iowa, which provides food to 389 partner agencies in 55 Iowa counties, was in desperate need of fresh produce to distribute to the hungry.

Newton Correctional Facility needed to teach offenders essential skills like problem solving, teamwork and responsibility. With 12 acres of extra land on site, the prison was uniquely situated to start a donation garden—using offenders' labor to plant, grow and harvest fresh fruits and vegetables.

"We need the produce, and they have the space," says Nathan Crozier, food sourcing specialist at the Food Bank of Iowa. "It's a natural partnership."

Joining Forces

The Newton Correctional Facility—a minimum- and medium-security prison located in Newton, Iowa—has been growing produce for its own

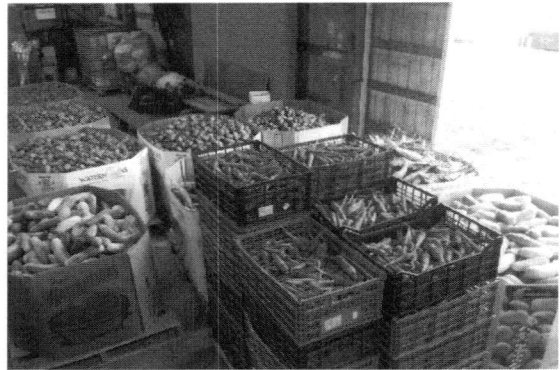

One morning's harvest from 12 acres at the Newton Correctional Facility offers much-needed produce for the Food Bank of Iowa's partner agencies.

use since it opened five decades ago.

Each year, offenders plant 12 acres of potatoes, onions, sweet corn and other Iowa staples. They harvest the crop and then clean, cook and serve meals to more than 1,300 men housed in the facility. In 2013, offenders working in the garden grew more than 86,000 pounds of food for the prison.

Because NCF had decades of experience growing food on their land, farming 12 more acres for the Food Bank of Iowa seemed like a simple next step. Still, the two institutions had to negotiate some tricky logistics—such as what and how much to grow, what equipment was needed and how to get the produce to the needy.

In the spring of 2012, the Food Bank of Iowa

provided the funds to help with initial setup costs (seeds, equipment and chemicals) to jump-start the second garden. Since then, the Fresh Produce Program, as it's known, has "grown by leaps and bounds," according to Aaron Baack, associate warden at NCF.

The two institutions work closely together, balancing the Food Bank of Iowa's needs with the produce that grows best on NCF land. Since the Food Bank of Iowa had no experience planning a large-scale garden, they relied on the correctional facility to provide crucial knowledge about agricultural techniques, produce varieties and equipment. But the free labor was the biggest gift of all.

In 2013, offenders worked in the Food Bank of Iowa garden for 2,800 hours, growing nearly 75,000 pounds of produce—carrots, cabbage, cucumbers, green peppers, watermelon and more. Using three small utility tractors and the hands and backs of motivated men, NCF was able to produce a harvest with a net value of more than $45,000—donated to people who would otherwise miss out on those essential vitamins and minerals.

"Overall, we were incredibly impressed to have the poundage that we did two drought years in a row," says Crozier of the 2012 and 2013 seasons.

Freshly Picked

Within a food-distribution system known for its cans and boxes, fresh fruits and vegetables are precious commodities for food banks. They're expensive, difficult to transport and hard to store. "Produce is not an easy thing to handle," says

Partners for Good

Interested in teaming up with a correctional facility to grow food for the hungry? Take these tips from the Food Bank of Iowa's Nathan Crozier and NCF's Aaron Baack.

Communicate. The Food Bank of Iowa and the Newton Correctional Facility are in constant contact.

Keep your eyes open. "Be aware of what you are getting yourself into in terms of workload and commitment," says Baack. Setting up a new garden requires a lot of labor.

Learn about agriculture. Even if your organization isn't doing the growing, it's best to learn as much as you can about the produce you'll be distributing and how it's produced, says Crozier.

Jump in, despite any doubts about logistics or hard work, Crozier advises. "What you are able to produce for the minimal cost you outlay is certainly worth it," adds Baack.

Crozier. "But it's what people need."

The Food Bank of Iowa is handing out more fruits and vegetables than ever before. In 2013, the nonprofit increased its distribution of fresh produce by 19 percent over the previous year. A huge portion of that came from the garden in Newton.

Every Wednesday during the growing season, depending on weather, the Food Bank of Iowa takes one of their trucks to NCF to load up hundreds of pounds of produce harvested by offenders the day before.

By the end of the day, those fruits and veggies are available to partner agencies all over the central portion of the state—food pantries, soup kitchens, homeless shelters, shelters for victims of domestic violence, and child and senior programs. Crozier says their partner agencies are "ecstatic" to receive the produce.

"The cost of produce is going through the roof," says Crozier. "Often items that are the cheapest are high in calories. So this produce is something those folks aren't getting normally."

Families on a tight budget can stretch their dollars more with unhealthy foods than with juicy fruit. So the produce grown in Newton is reaching people who may have lived on canned fruits and vegetables—or none at all—for years. Some pantries put out recipes incorporating seasonal produce for cooks unused to including them. The fresh greens make a huge nutritional difference for those individuals.

Learning Their Lesson

The Fresh Produce Program is a win-win for the state. In addition to providing nutritious, fresh food to low-income families, the program benefits the offenders, who learn marketable skills they can put to work after their release.

"Planning is first and foremost for them," says Baack. "Unfortunately, a lot of these folks didn't have the best planning skills when they came in. It was impulsive things that got them sent here."

Developing a 24-acre garden each spring takes a lot of planning. Rich Machin, an NCF staff member who supervises the garden, sits down with the workers at the beginning of each season to plot out the different items.

The offenders learn about agricultural techniques, water tables, safety equipment and tractor maintenance. They review a comprehensive garden handbook with step-by-step instructions for planting, growing and harvesting.

NCF refers to the knowledge and experience offenders gain in the garden as re-entry skills. In addition to the technical know-how, which may lead to higher wages or more responsibility after release, the offenders acquire skills that will help them succeed in any job, such as communication, teamwork, creative problem solving and a positive attitude.

"This prepares them to come to work," says Machin. "They get in the habit of coming to work."

One offender, whose initials are D.F., began his work assignment in March, attending a training class before beginning the planting season in mid-April. He loves being outside, which reminds him of the gardening he does back home. Still, he had to adjust to the team atmosphere that gardening on a large scale requires.

"I'm not a people person," he says. "Here, I work with a variety of people. I learn to be patient. The garden teaches us to be respectful of each other."

A Good Cause

Before the Food Bank of Iowa garden was created, working in the NCF garden was one of the most unpopular work assignments at the prison. Offenders chose maintenance, laundry, housekeeping or cafeteria duty over working outside in the harsh Iowa summers.

But once NCF started growing produce for the Food Bank of Iowa, that all changed overnight. Nearly 70 offenders applied for only 20 worker slots. Baack attributes the attitude change to the focus on doing good. "Being able to donate that harvest directly to the food bank—that's a good feeling."

In the dog days of August, offenders stay motivated to walk bean rows and pick cucumbers by reminding each other of the people they are feeding. "When the Food Bank of Iowa truck rolls up and we start loading produce, they just love that," says Baack. They even place guesses on the total poundage for that week to see who can come the closest.

D.F., especially, keeps hungry Iowans in mind while he is working. "I've been in a situation where I've been homeless," he says. "I've used food pantries. I appreciated the help. It's good to give back."

D.F. calls the partnership between the Food Bank of Iowa and NCF a "great idea." In addition to feeding people, the program instills an important lesson in the offenders, one that is applicable for all well-fed individuals.

"It teaches us that giving back to the community is not that hard," says D.F. "When we get out, we can do the same thing, if we choose to do it."

FOR MORE INFORMATION about building a partnership with the Food Bank of Iowa, visit **www.foodbankiowa.org**.

Spreading the Love

Start with an idea, get people involved, and you have Zestos, which every month feeds hundreds of people in northwest Iowa.

At the OK Café in Alton, Iowa, a landmark for decades in the main part of town, a chest freezer sits in the foyer, where the door is always unlocked. Rod and Jayne Hofmeyer and their volunteers put eight or 10 bags of groceries and tubes of meat in that freezer each day. By the next day, they're usually gone.

This arrangement shows how well the Hofmeyers understand Midwestern pride. "The bags are picked up by local people," Rod says, "who come under cloak of night if they need to."

The faith that inspired the unlocked foyer is the foundation for Zestos, which takes its name from a Greek word meaning "fervor of mind and zeal; to be zealous in the pursuit of good."

Run completely as a volunteer organization (Rod only recently started drawing a salary as the director), the nonprofit is committed to "caring for physical and spiritual needs with a special focus on those lacking even the basic necessities," Rod says.

For Rod and Jayne, it's an extension of their Christian faith. "We're a nondenominational Christian outreach organization. Everyone is welcome here."

Zestos began in 2008 when Rod was working at a local food-processing plant and saw how much food was being thrown away. After getting permission from his manager, he picked up the

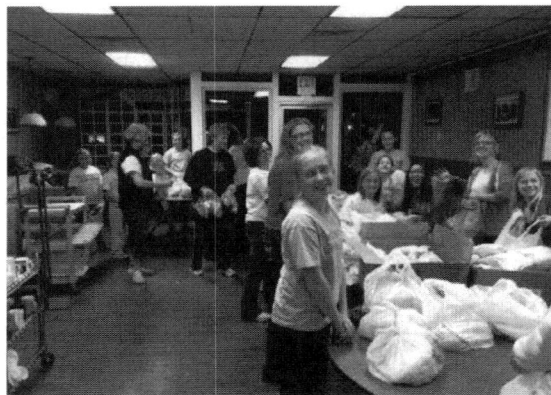

Volunteers with Zestos fill grocery bags of food to be distributed to food-insecure families at The Shepherd's Table gatherings.

food—sometimes eight or 10 pallets' worth of frozen, fully cooked meat products such as chicken nuggets and strips, hamburgers, chili and taco meat—and shared it with families in need. When the volume kept increasing, the Hofmeyers established Zestos.

"I picked up food on the second and fourth Tuesday of the month and found people with a freezer," Rod says. We used as much food as we could locally and took the overflow to Sioux City and shared it with a soup kitchen, and we put it in freezers in churches."

Before long, Zestos partnered with New Hope Church in Orange City to start a monthly banquet with a free meal and fellowship time, open to the public. Before people left, organizers

"OUR FIRST OFFICE WAS IN ORANGE CITY ON A HIGHWAY WITH A RUN-DOWN TRAILER PARK BEHIND IT. PEOPLE WENT FLYING DOWN THE HIGHWAY TO DO IMPORTANT THINGS—RIGHT PAST PEOPLE WHO WERE BROKE AND LIVING IN THE SHADOWS WITH EVERY KIND OF PROBLEM AND ISSUE. WE ARE SO BLIND TO A LOT OF STUFF GOING ON A FEW FEET AWAY."

asked if anyone had a friend or neighbor who needed a bag of groceries.

Word spread, and other churches contacted Zestos to arrange the same kinds of banquets and bags of groceries, called The Shepherd's Table, in their area.

Now, more than 14 churches in Orange City are involved in The Shepherd's Table, along with dozens of others in neighboring northwest Iowa communities. Donations come from businesses like Tyson Foods, Cloverleaf Cold Storage, Dean Foods, Fareway, Pizza Ranch, Hy-Vee, Casey's, Pizza Hut and The Dutch Bakery.

Volunteers pick up food on Monday and Friday, then package it up for bags of groceries. "The more people involved, the better," Rod says.

A couple of years ago, Zestos distributed fewer than 700 bags of food a month to people in northwest Iowa. In 2014, that number rose to 1,400, in addition to 400 or 500 boxes of bread and rolls.

"The increase is partly due to awareness of the program and bigger distribution," Rod says. "But there's more need in each town than before as well. The number of people struggling is growing."

The free meal and bag of groceries is a formula that works on a number of levels, Jayne says. "Through the years, we've struggled raising our family. A lot of times you're just one unexpected expense away from not having enough money, so we know there's a group of people just above the poverty line that really do have a need."

The offer of a bag of groceries circumvents the issue of pride, Jayne says. "We don't question why you're taking a bag of groceries. We just want to know you're going to use it. If you say it's for a neighbor but you're really using it, we don't care. We're just sharing what we have."

The Hofmeyers put their Zestos contact information—in English and Spanish—in every bag. "People call us for help, and we call a participating church in their area," Rod says. "We're like a unit working together."

Honor and Opportunity
Zestos expanded its services when it purchased the OK Café, which provides space for an office, meetings, food storage and Bible studies. It also has apartments upstairs, which means Zestos can help families in crisis transition to a more stable life.

While Rod was finalizing the building's purchase, he received a phone call. A woman with two children and a baby on the way was in a desperate situation. Her husband had been deported to Mexico, and she was destitute.

Volunteers from the Alton Reformed Church completed an "extreme apartment makeover," Rod says. "They redid the bathroom, painted and redid the kitchen, cabinets and all. A week later, we moved her in."

The woman and her children lived in the apartment for several months, until she was close to delivering her baby and walking up the steps

What One Church Can Do

This idea comes from Rod and Jayne Hofmeyer of Zestos, who told the story about the Alton Reformed Church in Alton, Iowa.

When the church's deacons received $1,000 in $50 gift cards from a local grocery store, they put the gift to good use. At the beginning of the service, Rod says, they drew numbers to see who in the congregation would get the cards.

The church members had to take the gift cards, and they had to *do* something with them. "They couldn't just give the card to someone who needed it," Rod says. "Instead, they had to buy food and cook a meal for a hungry family or something else—in other words, they had to take action."

On a following Sunday, the people who received a card came up to the front of the church and reported on how they'd used it. They all told how they'd ministered to a need.

"They weren't the people you usually see in front of the church," Rod says. "The common denominator was, they were all really excited about what they'd done. They got to live out their faith.

"People really do want to reach out, but they're not comfortable with it. It helps if you can get them to inch outside their comfort zone and do something like that."

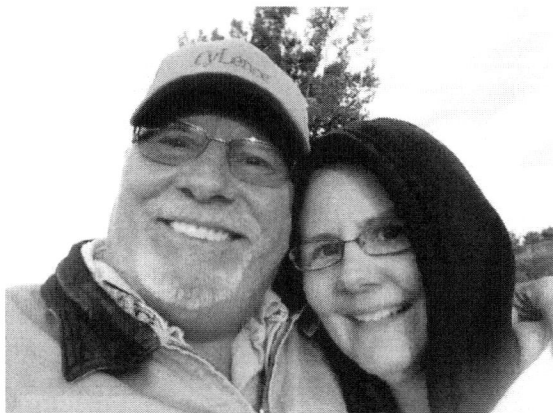
Rod and Jayne Hofmeyer of Zestos.

"WE DON'T QUESTION WHY YOU'RE TAKING A BAG OF GROCERIES. WE JUST WANT TO KNOW YOU'RE GOING TO USE IT."

to the second floor became a problem.

"We moved her into a mobile home," Rod says. "She owns it now." She's also working at the local hospital and working on her GED. "She interprets for us when we need an interpreter, and she helps package food and clean," Rod says. "She's made wonderful progress. It's just good, the way it's supposed to be."

Rod and Jayne have seen plenty of examples of the need in their community, and how local programs like Zestos can fill in the gaps.

"There are a lot of people who wouldn't expect to be in this situation at all," Rod says. "Maybe the husband and wife are both self-employed and the husband got injured and couldn't work."

Another example literally showed up at the doorstep of the OK Café.

"A woman pulled up to the café with six kids in an SUV," Rod says. "She had tears running down her cheeks because she was so humiliated. The bank had cut them off until they got their crop in, and they had no money to buy groceries."

The Zestos response was simple, and it characterizes everything you need to know about this organization.

"We loaded her up with food," Rod says. "What a wonderful honor and opportunity to help people like that."

FOR MORE INFORMATION about Zestos, visit **www.zestosinc.com**. Or email **zestosinc@gmail.com** or call **712/756-4456**.

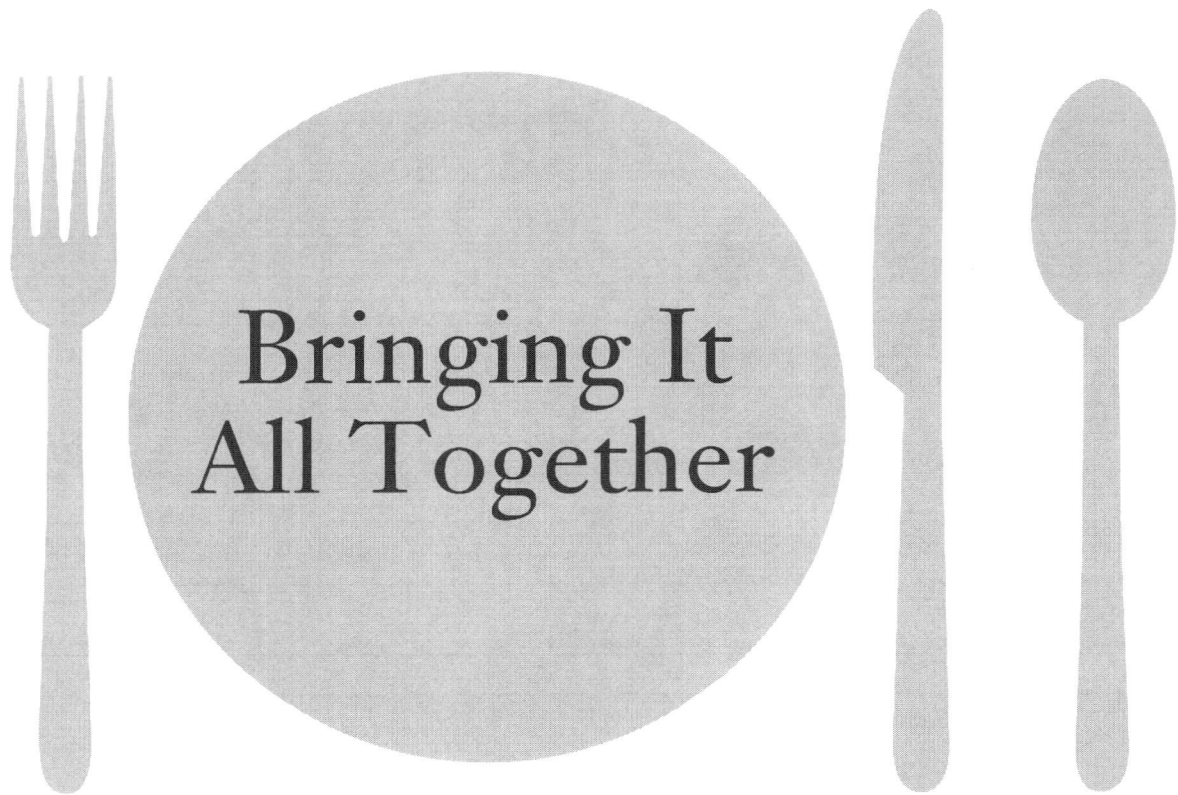

Bringing It
All Together

Growing Faith

For volunteers in the Faith and Grace Garden in West Des Moines, Iowa, feeding the hungry is a mission of biblical proportions.

We talked with Mark Marshall, founder, and Tim Goldman, garden coordinator, about the Faith and Grace Garden, a cooperative effort on land owned by St. Timothy's Episcopal Church and Covenant Presbyterian.

Q. How did the Faith and Grace Garden start?

MM: It was about 1997 or 1998, and I felt the need to start a small garden to bring in fresh vegetables, mainly for the elderly at the church here. Then eight or nine years ago I made a second garden where I planted probably 20 rows of peas and lettuce and radishes in between. That's the same time we started donating food to the Eddie Davis Community Center because we have a connection with them.

TG: It went this way up until the financial collapse in 2008, and then we became aware of more people needing food.

There was a meeting called Hope for the Hungry, and Mark went to speak about church

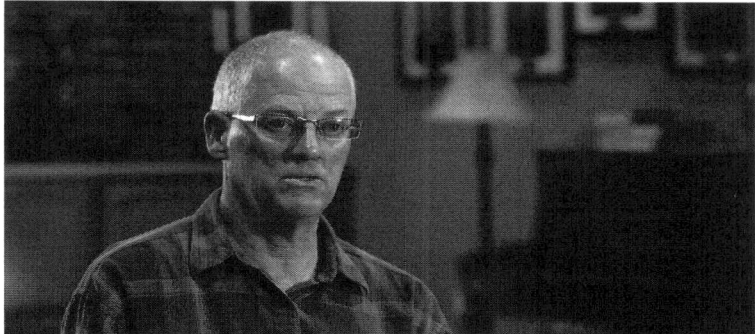

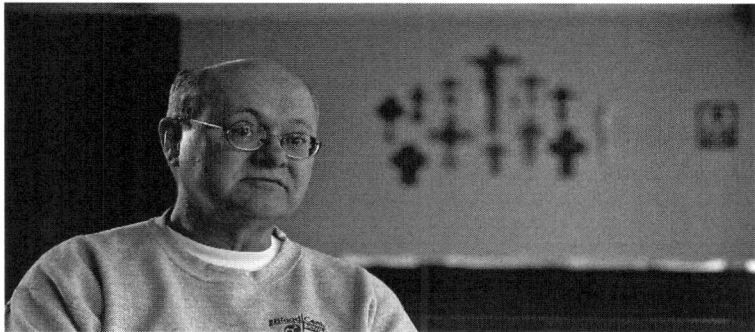

Mark Marshall, founder of the Faith and Grace Garden *(above)*. Timothy Goldman, garden coordinator *(below)*.

gardens and tell people how to get started. At that meeting, he ran into a fellow named Ray Meylor. Ray was with Isaac Walton League and informed Mark that he would come in with a plow and break up more ground if we wanted to have a donation garden. Mark took him up on that offer. In 2010 the garden grew from 2,500 square feet to 13,000 square feet. We had Ray in for the next few years, so in 2011 it was 27,000 square feet. In 2012 it was 38,000 square feet. And now if you throw in the flower beds—we have six of them in front of the garden—it's right at an acre in size.

"MORE AND MORE WE FIND THAT THE PEOPLE WE'RE FEEDING ALSO WANT TO COME TO THE GARDEN. THEY DON'T WANT TO JUST TAKE; THEY WANT TO GIVE, TOO."

Q. How much does the garden produce?

MM: In 2012 we donated 15,600 pounds. In 2013 it was close to 12,000 pounds.

TG: That food goes to the Des Moines Area Religious Council warehouse, where it then goes out to 14 different food pantries. In addition, we go to West Des Moines Human Services, Trinity Methodist, Cottage Grove Presbyterian Church (where they have a large Sudanese population), Children and Families of Iowa, and the battered women's shelter.

Q. When does the garden season start?

MM: Usually in mid January I start planting seeds for tomatoes and peppers. I have grow lights and heat mats in my basement, and I start 288 plants at a time. After two weeks, I start another batch. Last year, most of the school gardens around here got their plants from me. Then we start prepping the garden in March.

I call Ray Meylor, and he usually plows it up between the third week in March and the first of April. Then we're going at it again. In March, I'll usually go out and plant lettuce and spinach, radishes and peas. I've had peas peeking out of the snow before.

Q. How do you decide what to plant?

TG: We try to make sure we're growing food that's appropriate to the different populations that we serve. More and more we find that the people we're feeding also want to come to the garden. They don't want to just take; they want to give, too. So we'll have more people from different cultures and different ethnicities in the garden, and as they come in, we find they also have a lot to teach us.

Many of these people were subsistence farmers. They survived off of what they grew, and they bring in a completely different relationship with the land. We have some people who are trying to reconnect. But these people are already intimate with the land and are renewing their connection. They know how to very efficiently hoe around plants and get things done in a garden.

Q. Why are you so committed to the garden?

TG: It was February of 2010, and I hadn't been involved in the garden ministry at all, but I got to go and see where food from the garden had gone in the past.

I went to Trinity United Methodist Church on a Saturday morning. It was frigid outside, and the wind was blowing. We got there, and there was a line of people outside the door and down around the side of the building. There were a lot of people standing out in that weather.

I got to come to the front of the line and see what they were being given. What they were being given was two carrots, a quarter of a head of cabbage, and a can of stewed tomatoes. A lot of people without hats or gloves or heavy jackets on waited 45 minutes in frigid temperatures to get that food.

You could tell by the way they came through that line it was important to them. And I really couldn't believe we had that kind of a problem here in Des Moines. I was flabbergasted to see all the people, and it surprised me to see how little we could give them. I was told that some days it was even less.

"SUBURBAN CHURCHES SIT ON TWO, THREE, FOUR ACRES OF LAND, AND ALL THEY DO IS MOW IT. HERE WE ARE IN IOWA, WITH THE RICHEST LAND IN THE WORLD, AND WE COULD BE GROWING FOOD AND PROVIDING THE LOCAL AREA WITH FRESH PRODUCE."

MM: What motivates me to spend so much time here is the need for it. Since 2008 especially, there are a lot more unemployed people. When we first started doing this, there would be people crying when we'd bring them food. They were that happy to get it, to get fresh produce. It's a real sense of fulfillment to do it.

I grew up gardening, and I love to be out in the garden, so it's not really a job to me. I really love doing it, and it's extremely worthwhile.

Q. How is the garden making a difference?

TG: It's certainly making a difference in feeding people who need the food. It's definitely filling mouths and filling bellies.

I see it rippling out because maybe people who aren't working in their church garden see an opportunity to work at their school. We're seeing school gardens pop up.

And if you believe that people's spiritual lives are an underpinning of everything they do, we now see it not just in schools but in corporations.

Down the street from us, GuideOne has a large garden that their employees maintain, where they give away all the food. Things are starting up like that, so we see it spreading.

Q. What role does your faith play?

TG: We think the gospel message is unequivocal on our responsibility to feed people around us. And in doing that, every church has a role, and they can find different ways to address it. For us it's a garden.

We've been very pleased through the efforts of the community that we've grown from about 4,000 pounds a year to almost 16,000. That's been due to the help of our neighbors next door, churches across the way, businesses that are in this area and a lot of people we don't even know who will lend tools to us, seeds...all sorts of things. People seem to be concerned about hunger and want to resolve it.

Q. How much of a need do you see?

TG: One thing we're finding is that we'll have people we just find in the garden, asking if they can pick some food. And before long they're explaining about their lost job or the health issue that their family member has.

They'll say, "I just was at the grocery store, and I was only able to get one or two things, and I really need something for tonight." And they pick a few things and leave. It's so great to hand them a plastic bag and say, "Fill it up." They're so appreciative.

They can get into a car that looks as good as yours or mine and drive away because they recently lost a job. People live paycheck to paycheck that we don't always recognize, and they can be in great trouble in a relatively short space of time.

Q. What kind of volunteer staff does it take to keep the garden going?

MM: Someone's in the garden at least six days a week, and seven's not uncommon. I'm here six days a week, and then Tim is also here a good four days a week.

Then we've tried to recruit other adults to help. There are Dowling Catholic High School students—especially in the spring, when there's anywhere from six to twenty students here. On a typical night there'll be twenty people here. And then on Sundays too. Tim usually takes Saturday mornings, and I take Sundays.

It's going to be slow. I'm not going to lie. It's tough in the beginning. You spend lots of hours here hoping to get volunteers, but it gets better every year.

Q. What message do you have for other churches?

MM: What I would like to say to other churches is what I've said at the Hope for the Hungry conferences. Suburban churches especially sit on two, three, four acres of land, and all they do is mow it. Here we are in Iowa, with the richest land in the world, and we could be growing food and providing the local area with fresh produce. You could be growing food that tastes wonderful and help eliminate the carbon footprint of having food brought in by truck. So if every church could just find a couple of dedicated members to undertake the leadership in getting the garden going, I think they would find plenty of help.

Q. Are more churches getting involved?

TG: I think you're seeing a lot of response locally. I know when we started looking at this about three years ago, there were three churches in the Des Moines area that had gardens on their property. I think there are 15 or 16 now, so it's grown a lot in the last few years. And there are several more that are looking at it.

Some churches that have looked at having a garden have said they don't have the land for it, but they do send people out to the other churches that have gardens, so we have a wonderful synthesis going on here.

In our gospel, we're told to feed the hungry, to care for the sick and to visit the prisoner. I think it's in the gospel of Luke about every sixth line, and in the gospel of Matthew about every eighth line, so it's a strong commandment that we're all given to feed the hungry.

Q. Would this kind of church garden work in smaller towns?

MM: I think the difference it could make in a small community would be even greater than in Des Moines. You're talking half a million people in Des Moines. If you took a town of 10,000 or less people, and one or two churches in that town were to put one to two acres into a garden, they could literally supply the whole town with fresh produce.

Q. Are there ways non-gardeners can help?

TG: Anyone who wants to address the hunger issue certainly can do that. They can do it with their time or with their money. They may have garden tools they're no longer using. They may just want to come and sit in the garden and help us supervise children. So anybody who wants an opportunity to serve in a garden is certainly able to do that.

Q. What's the key to making a church garden work?

MM: If twenty people are out here for one hour, that's like me coming ten times for two hours. Numbers are the whole key when it comes to solving the problem. It takes a small effort if enough people are willing to donate just a little bit of time. And if we had ten churches with a one-acre garden, that would be 100,000 pounds of vegetables. It's just a matter of the commitment to do it.

FOR MORE INFORMATION visit **www.growthefood.org**.

What the Faith and Grace Garden Volunteers Are Saying

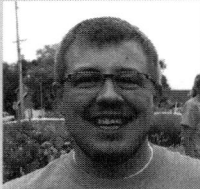

John Charbonneaux
Sr. Client Service Associate
with Principal Financial Group
Retirement Investor Services

Principal employees volunteer all over the community. The company is really great about giving us volunteer time off. They give us eight hours a year to come out and do these different projects and give back to the community.

I think we may take things for granted. We go home and flip the lights on and have a warm meal to heat up and you don't think about hunger, but there are people in our community who are going hungry every day.

So if I have the means to come out and the physical ability to help somebody else put food on their table, I think it's important. If we could all pull together, it would be a much nicer world.

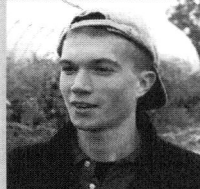

Jacob Luksan
Student, Dowling Catholic
High School in West
Des Moines, Iowa

I got introduced to Intro to Entre-preneurship at Dowling, which prepared me for this class, which is directly involved with Faith and Grace Garden.

It teaches you how to own a business. And when you own a business, you have to tend to it and care for it just like a garden. That's the main priority we have here—to tend it and take care of it.

When we go to the different charities and deliver the produce by hand, it's amazing to see the people's different reactions and how polite they are and how they actually need this food.

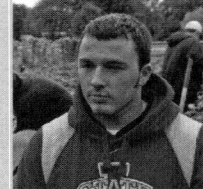

Nick Topping
Student, Dowling Catholic
High School in West
Des Moines, Iowa

This garden can impact the community by helping those in the metro area. It grows the produce, and we give it to the food pantries in the Des Moines area. Also, it can help by teaching the kids at Dowling how to work in a business setting and how to work in a group.

You learn a lot about working with your hands and being in little teams and getting a main goal accomplished together.

It's something that any school could do. Any schools could help out here, and they could help out at other gardens around the area.

Shopping for Seeds

Mark Marshall, founder of the Faith and Grace Garden in West Des Moines, has been starting seeds for his church and school gardens for more than 15 years. Here's his list of favorite varieties and vendors, based on getting the best yield for the best price.

American Seed Company
(www.AmericanSeedCo.com)

Pole Beans: Blue Lake Stringless

Bush Beans: Tenderette, Roma II, Royal Burgundy, Slenderwax

Lima Beans: Fordhook 242, Burpee's Improved

Soybeans: Vinton 81

Beets: Detroit Dark Red, Golden Detroit, Lutz Green Leaf

Cabbage: Red Acre, Golden Acre Y.R., Pak Choi

Cantaloupe: Hale's Best, Honey Dew

Watermelon: Black Diamond, Crimson Sweet

Sweet Corn: Incredible SE, Sugar Baby SE

Bay Farm Services, Inc.
(www.mainstreetseedandsupply.com)

Peas: Thomas Laxton, Oregon Sugar Pod

Pole Beans: Kentucky Wonder (yellow)

George's Plant Farm (www.tatorman.com)

Sweet Potatoes: Georgia Jet

Des Moines Feed & Garden

Potato Seed: Red Pontiac, Yukon Gold, Kennebec

Onion Sets: red, white & yellow

Other favorite seeds, saved from year to year:

Tomatoes: Big Beef, Roma, San Marzano, Mortgage Lifter

Sweet Peppers: Cal Wonder, Canary Bell, Chocolate Bell, Purple Bell, Orange Bell, Marconi

Hot Peppers: Anaheim, Big Jim, Jalapeno, Jabañero, Serrano, Thai, Poblano, Hot Pasilla, Mulato

Cucumbers: Straight 8

Summer Squash: Dark Green & Golden Zucchini

Winter Squash: Green Hubbard, Table Queen, Burgess Buttercup, Spaghetti

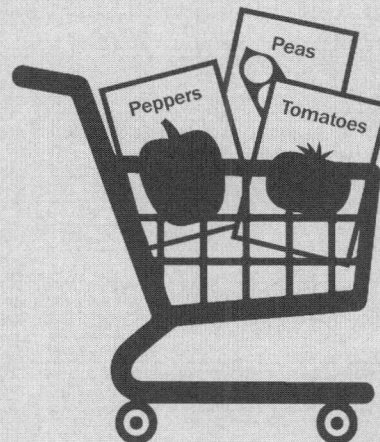

A TIP FROM MARK MARSHALL: "Ask the people who receive the food what they'd like you to plant, such as a particular pepper for Mexican mole sauce."

A Land to Call Home

Refugees from countries all over the world feed themselves and others through the rich Iowa soil.

A few years ago, Nicholas Wuertz was taking a typical drive across Iowa. Bored by the routine scenery, he turned toward the people in the backseat. He found them wide-eyed, silent with astonishment. As far as they could see, the rolling hills were producing food. Refugees primarily from Asia or Africa, they had never been outside Des Moines since first touching down at the airport.

"This is what we know how to do," they said of the corn rows and the acres of soybeans. "How do we get some of this land?" Iowa, with its bitter winds and mystifying white winters, suddenly seemed familiar. Iowa was a little bit like home.

"Most of the people coming to the United States right now are from agrarian backgrounds," says Hilary Burbank, supervisor of the Global Greens program at Lutheran Services in Iowa (LSI). "It wasn't so much a job as a lifestyle. It was the way they raised their families."

Wuertz is now program director for LSI's Refugee Community Services program. And the travelers that day were refugees served by LSI in Des Moines, on their way to a conference. When they returned, fresh with new ideas, they worked with LSI employees to begin the Global Greens program, connecting refugees

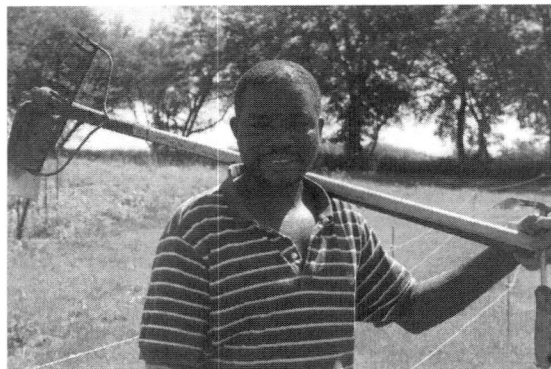

Charles Bizimana uses a hoe with an extra long blade, a favorite tool of the farmers from Africa and Asia. The refugees have shared agricultural knowledge with their Iowa neighbors.

with community gardens.

Four years later, about 150 refugees grow their own food in 11 gardens throughout the Des Moines metro area—some on land provided by the city and others on private property.

Many of these newcomers to the state would otherwise not be able to afford the high-priced fruits and vegetables available in stores. A garden means they can feed their families plenty of nutritious food and their native crops.

"There was a core group of people who really wanted to move onto larger land and sell their food as a business," says Burbank. Thanks to

A GARDEN MEANS THEY CAN FEED THEIR FAMILIES PLENTY OF NUTRITIOUS FOOD AND THEIR NATIVE CROPS.

the Valley Community Center, which provided space on their property, LSI was able to create a four-acre incubator farm in West Des Moines, where 26 refugee families grow produce to sell to the community. The goal is to prepare the farmers to transition to their own land in three to five years.

"They know things instinctively because they have farmed all their lives," says Zach Couture, farm associate at the Global Greens Farm. From the 26 families, eight advanced market farmers receive intensive training in agricultural methods, record-keeping and marketing.

Anyone growing food at the farm can sell produce at farmer's markets each week in the summer. The market accepts SNAP and WIC (Women, Infants and Children) benefits, which allows other refugees and low-income families to purchase the healthy produce, including greens and herbs they ate in their home countries.

Although the sales provide the struggling farmers with much-needed income, the Global Greens program is about more than financial security. "The heart of it overrides the monetary side of it," says Burbank. "Having a place, having land, is really important, especially for these folks, who lost their land."

At Home in Iowa

In 1975, Governor Robert Ray answered the international call to accept 1,200 Laotian refugees

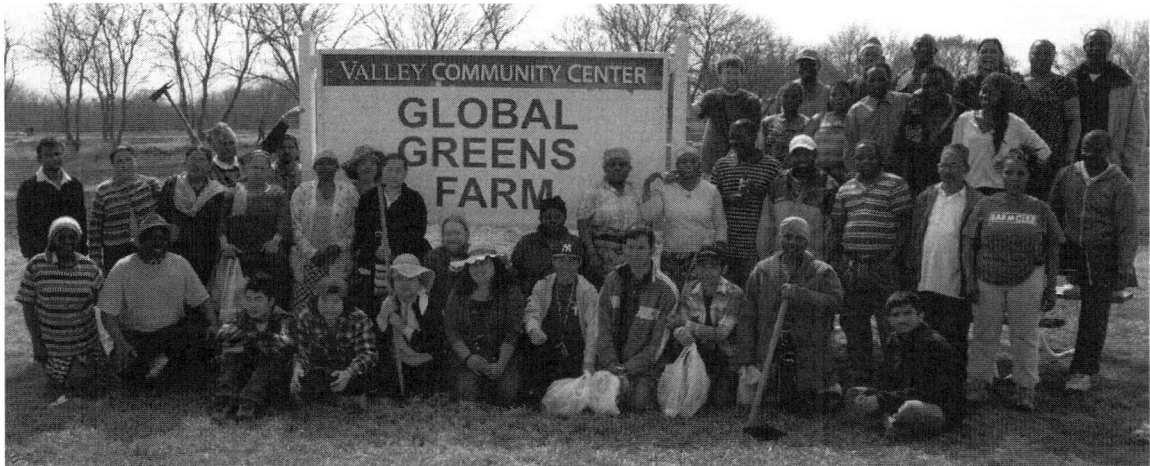

Twenty-six refugee families grow food for themselves and their customers at the Global Greens Farm in West Des Moines, on land provided by the Valley Community Center.

who were imperiled by the end of the Vietnam War. Since then, Iowa has been a leader in refugee resettlement, offering a new homeland to more than 30,000 refugees over four decades.

LSI Refugee Community Services provides a variety of assistance to refugees, including ESL and work-readiness classes. Currently, many refugees are coming to Iowa from Burma (Myanmar) and Bhutan in Asia and Burundi and Rwanda in central Africa. All these countries are primarily agrarian, and most of the refugees have a personal history with farming.

The refugees who grow food in community gardens or on the Global Greens Farm spend less money on groceries and eat healthier food. The savings allows them to pay for other necessities like clothing, school supplies and utilities. By providing many of their own meals, they are able to skip visits to food pantries and soup kitchens, taking the strain off an already-stretched food distribution system.

The program has other benefits, too. Refugees are in danger of isolation within their new communities, but gardening brings them into social contact with others. Connection with the soil can bring about emotional healing for past traumas, reminding them of cultural traditions back home. The farmers often bring multiple generations out to weed and harvest, and the children learn about their home culture and the basics of growing food.

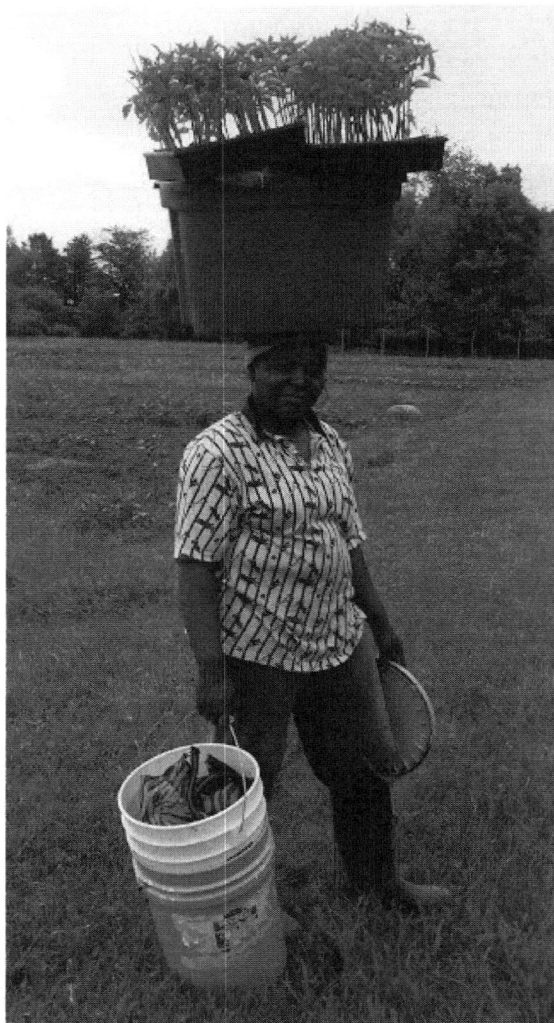

Jacqueline, a refugee farmer from Burundi, saves time by using her head as she works her plot at the Global Greens Farm.

"Farming gives a sense of pride for people," says Couture. "They feel they are accomplishing something."

Down on the Farm

At the Global Greens Farm, the refugees cultivate dozens of Iowa staples: tomatoes, onions, corn, peppers, strawberries, all Certified Naturally Grown.

"We plant American food," Arcade Nsangayezu, a refugee from Burundi, says proudly. "It's good to learn how to plant food from everywhere." But he and his dad, Simon Bucumi, are eager to have their customers try renga renga, a favorite green from central Africa that tastes like spinach and is rich in iron and calcium. "We like to share our culture with Americans, mix American culture with Burundi."

Among the usual suspects in the garden plots, the refugees also grow unexpected produce: sweet potato leaves, African eggplants, Napa cabbage, lemongrass and wapato, or Indian potato. "I like seeing and trying

Recipe for a Refugee Garden

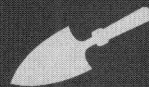

Refugees are perfect candidates for community gardens. They often need the food, and many have agricultural backgrounds. Instead of feeding refugees with a one-time donation, consider helping them feed themselves for years to come.

Contact local food pantries. Since pantries serve refugee populations, they can tell you where to find the newcomers in your neighborhood.

Approach social service agencies. Just like food pantries, these agencies can identify the leaders of the ethnic communities you need to meet.

Form a partnership. Refugees are often isolated in public housing. It's important to get them involved in the project from the start. "Come to the poor," says Tim Goldman, coordinator of the Faith and Grace Garden in West Des Moines. "Don't just hand them a basket of this or that. Get to know the commonality between you."

Start with a community garden. Hilary Burbank of LSI advises helping refugees grow their own food first before selling it. Expand slowly, as the gardeners are ready.

Know your markets. If and when you are prepared to sell the produce, pinpoint customers first. Do you want to focus on the refugee community and accept SNAP benefits? Or should you sell at the higher-priced farmer's markets already established? "The refugees can grow the food," says Burbank, "but the biggest barrier is getting it out there."

crops I didn't know anything about before," says Couture.

As teacher and mentor, he focuses on weed and pest management, the toughest aspects of agriculture. "They are really good at growing food," Couture says of the refugee farmers. "They know how to water, weed and till. From the North American point of view, we want to add a little bit more science into it. We want to improve their efficiency."

The refugee farmers don't have an easy job, growing food by hand and then finding customers in a new country. Burbank describes them as "incredibly hard-working." She says that, despite the labor, there is always a great spirit out in the field.

Simon Bucumi and his son are eager to grow, obtaining more customers and more land. They are always thinking about the future. Still, they cherish every moment of this experience. "When we sell our food, it's like a new day!" says Bucumi.

Business School

Minah Yang Somsanith, farm marketing specialist at LSI, is responsible for preparing the advanced market farmers for the American business world. She focuses on record-keeping and marketing, emphasizing expenses and income. She also teaches them how to identify potential customers and stand out at a market. Every month,

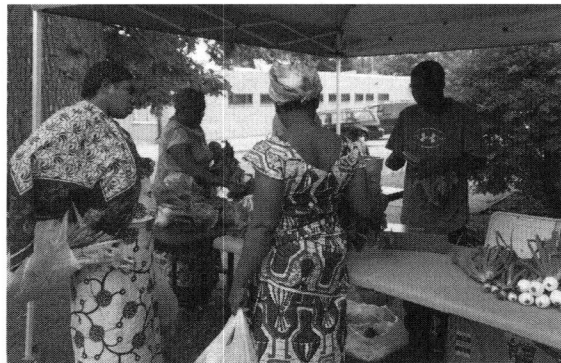

Shoppers, both refugees and native Iowans, purchased refugee-grown produce this summer at the Saturday farmer's market at Lutheran Services in Iowa.

she meets with each family one-on-one to go over harvest and sales numbers and address any problems that come up.

Somsanith is a child of refugees, so she knows the pitfalls that can face those new to English and to this country. "I know I wouldn't be who I am without the help that we received," says Somsanith. "I just want to make sure that I can impact their lives as much as others have impacted mine."

A Two-Way Street

In the end, the refugees at LSI impact the native Iowans just as much. In his home garden, Couture grows his vegetables the way the refugees taught him—in short perpendicular rows. But the most important lessons are intangible.

THE GLOBAL GREENS PROGRAM IS FEEDING PEOPLE WHO LACK ENOUGH HEALTHY FOOD—BOTH THE FARMERS THEMSELVES AND THEIR NEIGHBORS IN NEED. IN SEARCH OF NEW LAND, THE REFUGEES CAME TO IOWA AND FOUND THEY HAD SOMETHING IN COMMON WITH THE PEOPLE ALREADY HERE.

"We have a lot to learn from people who have been really close to the soil and had to depend on it for all their food," says Tim Goldman, coordinator at the Faith and Grace Garden, where refugees come to work.

Faith and Grace grew more than 11,000 pounds of produce in 2013 to donate to food pantries, domestic violence shelters and churches that serve the undocumented. They have hundreds of volunteers, including 15 refugees from LSI. *(See more about the Faith and Grace Garden on page 91.)*

Goldman notices that the refugees have a reverence for the land. Some take off their shoes in the garden; others sing. Working becomes a social time, a chance to build community. The refugees have also taught Goldman about his own garden, pointing out different edible weeds *(see sidebar, page 105).*

"That whole connection with each other and with the soil is something that, if you watch people in the garden over time, you see a lot of us from the West have simply lost," says Goldman. "We are paying more attention to our devices than

to creation." The refugees, he says, can teach us about nature just by being there.

Reconciling Refugees

Refugees find new homes all across Iowa, inspiring other communities to connect with them. After buying land to build a new church, members of New Disciples of Cedar Rapids felt that God was calling them to start a garden there.

The congregation funded an analysis of their neighborhood and learned that one of the top five needs was adequate healthy food. They decided to bring together the diverse populations of the southwest side of the city in an effort to grow nutritious food for those who needed it.

The church termed the project a reconciliation garden, with the goal of bringing together people from different racial, cultural and socioeconomic backgrounds. One of those groups included refugees from Central Africa, specifically Burundi, Zambia and the Democratic Republic of the Congo.

Stasia Fine, pastor of New Disciples, learned that some of the families from Africa dislike American food because they see it as unhealthy.

But they couldn't afford expensive fruits and vegetables in stores.

"Fresh food is really important to them," says Fine. "But not all food pantries have fresh food." Now, any produce the refugees and other gardeners don't take gets donated to the local pantry.

Inspired by the needs of the neighborhood, the garden is devoted to the sharing of food. All the seeds are donated, and anyone can plant food or harvest it. The garden is sponsored by the Blue Zones Project (**www.iowa.bluezonesproject. com**), whose mission is to help communities live longer, healthier lives.

One of the major initiatives is eating healthy, which is especially important for refugees and other low-income populations who don't have as much access to fresh produce. That goal resonates with the Africans, who come to the garden before and after work every day.

"I don't think that the people who have grown up in the United States for several generations put that same value on fresh food as our families from Africa do," says Fine.

Due to their generosity, the New Disciples congregation has given hungry refugees the chance to not only eat well, but to grow their own food in a way that can sustain them for years. Fine says their efforts were guided by their faith story in the Bible, which is no stranger to the concept of refugees.

"The families from Africa are our brothers and sisters," says Fine. "They are not foreigners. They are part of our family."

Growth Spurt

The people at LSI have come to think of the refugees as family, too, even though they come from all across the world. The staff has seen families grow and achieve their goals. In a way, the Global Greens program has grown up with the farmers, expanding each time the refugees pushed them for more land.

The Global Greens program is feeding people who lack enough healthy food—both the farmers themselves and their neighbors in need. In search of a new land, the refugees came to Iowa and found they had something in common with the people already here.

The idea of growing food, of feeding yourself and the hungry—that connects all Iowans, those born here or thousands of miles away. Iowans can't escape the agricultural landscape all around them—the farmer's markets, the sweet corn stands, the backyard gardens, the rows of corn beneath an endless sky.

"Everyone here has a farming background," says Somsanith of both the Iowans and the refugees. "We are all connected by farming."

FOR MORE INFORMATION about the Global Greens program and the refugee programs at Lutheran Services in Iowa, visit **www.lsiowa.org**.

Edible Weeds

One day in the Faith and Grace Garden, Tim Goldman found a group of refugees picking sacks of weeds. He thought the pickers were going to throw them out; instead, they took the weeds home to eat.

Since then, the refugees have taught Goldman about many edible weeds, and now he makes sure they get to people who will eat them, whether the refugee gardeners themselves or food pantries serving immigrant populations.

"In areas where it's arid or there is poor soil quality, their garden vegetables are our weeds," says Goldman. "Weeds are much tougher and easier to grow than some of the things we call food sources."

Check with a horticultural expert before eating or donating weeds like these from your yard.

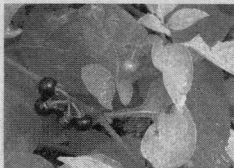

Black Nightshade (*solanum nigrum*) sounds menacing, but the toxicity varies greatly. In central Africa, the leaves—high in vitamin A—are boiled twice with tomatoes to make a beloved staple. Others eat the berries or bake them into pies. However, there are many different varieties of this weed, and it's difficult for amateurs to tell the edible from the poisonous. Avoid eating the wild weed, and make sure you can trust the source of any cultivated nightshade.

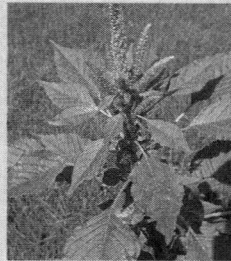

Common lambsquarters (*Chenopodium album*) is a summer annual that can adapt to nearly any environment, making it a common backyard weed across the U.S. A cousin to quinoa, lambsquarters is high in vitamins A and C, calcium, potassium and iron. Often compared to spinach, some say it's even tastier than the popular green, especially when sautéed in olive oil. Goldman says refugees working in the Faith and Grace Garden would pick the weed instead of taking home lettuce.

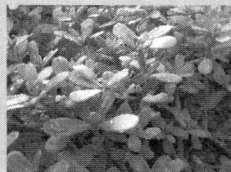

Pigweed (*Amaranthus*) is a troublesome variety of weed for farmers across Iowa. The plant originated in the Americas and then spread across the globe. Known as renga renga in Burundi and grown as a crop throughout the continent, it's Africa's most nutritious vegetable, with greens rich in iron, calcium, niacin, carotene and vitamins A and C. The leaves can be boiled like spinach or eaten raw in a salad.

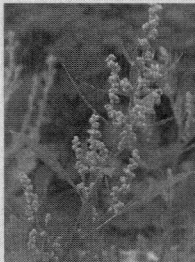

Purslane (*Portulaca oleracea*) first emerged in India and Persia before spreading to the Americas. With succulent and yellow flowers, the plant thrives in both fertile and arid soils, making it one of the most frequently reported weeds in the world. Hailed for its crunchiness and subtle lemon flavor, purslane leaves can be put on salads or sandwiches, thrown into pesto sauces or used to thicken soup or stew. With six times more vitamin E than spinach and seven times more beta-carotene than carrots, purslane is more nutritious than some of our common veggies.

Starting the Conversation

Want to change the way your community addresses hunger?
It all starts with a dialogue.

We talked with Angie Tagtow, co-founder of the Iowa Food Systems Council and convener of the Iowa Food Access and Health Work Group, about the ways communities can start to change policy and feed the hungry close to home.

Q. How did you get interested in hunger issues?
A. I'm a public health dietitian by training and spent many years working with the Iowa Department of Public Health and the Women, Infants and Children (WIC) program.

WIC is a federally funded discretionary program that provides nutrition services and education to women who are pregnant or breast-feeding, or have infants and children up to the age of five. In addition to providing a prescribed food package, WIC provides nutrition education and referral sources for those families.

That's where I got my very first taste, if you will, of issues of food insecurity and hunger

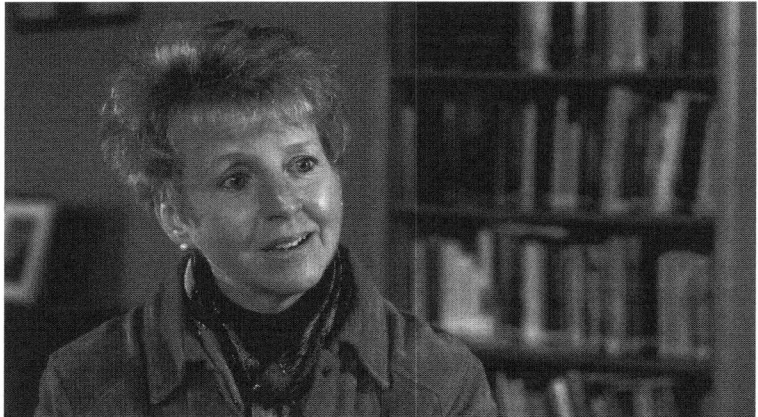

Angie Tagtow, co-founder of the Iowa Food Systems Council.

in the state of Iowa. One of my responsibilities with that job was to assess the extent of food insecurity among WIC participants. And I had the opportunity of working with Mark Nord at the USDA and developing the process for assessing food insecurity among WIC participants. The fascination and interest grew from there.

My very first day working with the Iowa Department of Public Health, I was put on the road with a colleague to visit a clinic in northwest Iowa. I distinctly remember walking through the clinic with a woman

who had come in with five of her 11 or 12 children. She was really struggling to get through the clinic, not being able to remember things and not having the things to take care of her kids that day.

At the end of clinic, I found out she lived on a farm. I was very perplexed at the fact that this was a farm family that couldn't make ends meet and put food on their own table.

This was really astounding for me that that happens here in Iowa. Iowa, literally the heart of America's breadbasket, has rising rates of food insecurity when we

"WE NEED TO CHANGE OUR PERCEPTION ABOUT LOW-RESOURCE INDIVIDUALS…THE MAJORITY OF PEOPLE WHO GO TO EMERGENCY FEEDING SITES ARE EMPLOYED INDIVIDUALS, BUT THE SALARY THEY MAKE ISN'T ABLE TO MEET THEIR NEEDS."

are one of the leading agricultural producers in the country. That really perplexed me.

From there on, I started to be critical about what was happening around me in Iowa and why there was such a dichotomy between what's happening—literally—in the fields around me vs. what was happening in WIC. Our agricultural system doesn't necessarily support our nutrition system, and our agricultural policies don't necessarily support nutrition policies in this country.

Q. Did you learn other things about hunger in Iowa through the WIC program?

A. Yes. As a dietitian, not only was it my responsibility to interpret federal policy for implementation at the local level, but also to assist our local agencies in providing the best services they could for the people coming to see them.

I always was surprised at the challenges that our front-line staff witnessed day to day. Going out and doing these WIC clinic visits, I continued to be amazed at the families coming in and in need of services. Most of them were working. Most of them of course had children because they were involved in the WIC program. They kind of dispelled a lot of the perceptions we may have of low-income Iowans.

These are hard-working folks who just don't have the resources to meet all of their financial needs—food being one of them. I grew to really appreciate the hard work that it took to take care of a young family when you have limited resources to do so.

In the ten years I worked with the state WIC program, that never changed.

We really need to change the perception about low-resource individuals in this state and in this country. The majority of people who are enrolled in the food and nutrition assistance programs or who visit emergency feeding sites are employed individuals. The problem is that the salary they make isn't enough to meet their and their family's needs. So at the crux of the issue of hunger and food insecurity is the issue of poverty and household income. We can't have a conversation about hunger without having a deep conversation about poverty and income in this country.

Q. Are there other contributing factors to

hunger and food insecurity?

A. Iowa really is a paradox. The fact is that we dedicate 30 million acres in this state to agriculture—that's 86 percent of our landscape—and the focus on most of that land is: how can we grow more per acre? So we've been able to increase yields over the last 10 years on those fields. But as we see rising yields in our agricultural landscape, we're also seeing a rising need for food and nutrition assistance and emergency feeding.

We have 400,000 Iowans who don't know where their next meal is coming from. How can we, in a very rich agricultural state, also have rising rates of hunger? That is the biggest paradox. So, to get at the conversation on the rising rates of food insecurity, we have to look at household incomes. We have to look at and evaluate what people are making in order to sustain a family.

One of the first things that happens on a household level when food budgets start to thin down is that families look at food and nutrition assistance programs and emergency feeding programs. We really need to evaluate that.

But it's not necessarily just livable wages for all Iowans. We need to look at what's happening in the community as well. Those who are making livable and sustainable wages are able to support a more vital and vibrant community. They go hand in hand.

Again, we have this paradox with what's going on around us and with what's happening with our neighbors and our family members. How do we look at one to support the other?

The other paradox that exists in this situation is: What does Iowa grow? What do not only low-resource individuals but all Iowans need to ensure nutrition security? We have food insecurity, but are we working to achieve nutrition security as well?

When we start to dissect what's grown here in this state and parallel that to the USDA's My Plate, we find that Iowa agriculture falls very short of meeting nutrition needs in this state. Our definition of food insecurity from an individual household level now expands to a discussion about food and nutrition security at a state level.

Does and can Iowa agriculture provide enough nutrition for the 3 million people who live here? The potential is there. But do we have the political will to change agricultural policies that best support nutrition policies?

Q. What are the issues of access to food?

A. In rural areas what we've seen in a retail environment is a lot of consolidation within our grocery and supermarket chains. We've seen our Mom and Pop or smaller grocery stores have to leave a community only to be replaced by a mega store or grocery store that might be in a nearby town. So distance to travel to access healthy foods is a big consideration when we have this discussion.

In urban areas it may be a

family that doesn't have transportation and has to rely on public transportation. In a rural setting it might mean traveling into the nearest town to a convenience store to get their groceries, for the week perhaps, and then occasionally traveling to a town 30 or 40 miles away that may have a full-fledged grocery market with a diverse array of foods.

So we have what we call food deserts in both urban and rural areas. That's a new set of data we have access to that can easily be incorporated into community discussions.

Q. How does hunger impact society?
A. Hunger is a problem directly related to poverty and income. Hunger is not just a problem of the government, not just a problem of unemployed people, not just a problem of those in the lowest socioeconomic class. Hunger affects all of us.

One of simplest steps we can take is to begin the conversation.

Start to find out more about what's happening in your community that is directly related to hunger. Bring people together to have those conversations. Dig up the data.

The next step is to identify the extent of the problem, then identify solutions. Begin having conversations with policy makers in your community, city council members, your neighbors, and let them know what's happening. The conversations have to start to move in that direction.

Here in the Midwest, we have the issue of pride. So often we don't boast about our accomplishments, nor do we talk about the challenges we have. Many families don't let others know they're struggling. So often hunger and food insecurity becomes a very hidden topic in communities.

Putting a face on those who are struggling brings a whole new dimension into this conversation. If you know somebody who might be struggling to put food on the table, you're more apt to

do something about it.

Q. What would you like to see in Iowa in the next five years?
A. Iowa should not have hunger. In the richest agricultural state in this country, no Iowan should be hungry. In the next five years, I would hope we would have much more alignment with what's happening on our farmland and what's happening on our plates.

Another thing I'd wish for is addressing the root of hunger in Iowa. At the state level we have not had an in-depth conversation about poverty and ensuring that all Iowans have a livable wage.

Q. Why does this matter to you personally?
A. If citizens are not healthy, communities will not be able to realize their optimal potential. We have to have healthy natural resources and a healthy food system to ensure the well-being of all Iowans.

FOR MORE INFORMATION, visit **www. iowafoodsystemscouncil.org**.

Conversation Starters

Building a coalition to address hunger in your community doesn't take special credentials or titles. Here are a few tips from Angie Tagtow to help you take the first steps.

1. Find out what's already happening in your community.

"Maybe the best place for these conversations to start is with your civic organizations. Check in with your county to see what exists in your community and what can be capitalized on. That's an excellent venue for starting."

2. Look for community transformation grants.

"One of the exciting things happening right now is community transformation grants.

"Counties are looking at how they can make more healthful communities by pulling together food

systems stakeholders: folks from university extension, the medical community, farmers, processors and Department of Natural Resources staff.

"They're assessing food access in the community, even beyond those who are participating in food-emergency feeding programs.

"Where does the whole community access food? Where are the closest grocery stores? Are more people going to convenience stores or perhaps liquor stores for food? Engage these stakeholders to come up with viable solutions."

3. Introduce more school gardens.

"School gardening has brought a new dimension to the curriculum and food service. It brings new dimensions to community activities through gardening alone."

4. Evaluate the built environment.

"Look at built environments that support healthy living. Look at bike trails, hiking paths and other recreational things that have been established and are identified with what will make your community healthy."

5. Talk about ways you can help one another.

"Some of the most

successful initiatives and movements have started at someone's kitchen table. Something started and became a groundswell among more people in that community. With just the beginning of that conversation, we can move forward with instrumental changes. But it takes the conversation to start that. It requires neighbors to talk to neighbors, co-workers to talk to co-workers. We need to get our youth in on this conversation.

"The critical conversation is key. We come from a heritage in Iowa where we step forward and help our neighbor. The best thing we can do is to help our neighbors today."

The Commitment of a Lifetime

For writer Rachel Vogel Quinn, helping the hungry is part of her family's history. In her words, here's the story of her grandfather and the origins of his lifelong mission.

Bartholomew "Bud" Vogel began life stocking shelves in his parents' general store in Andalusia, Illinois, a small town just across the Mississippi from Iowa. At the end of his life, he was stocking the shelves of local food pantries and the River Bend Foodbank. As his wife Kay loved to joke, "He sure didn't come very far."

In Andalusia, the Vogel general store served as a lifeline for the entire community during the Great Depression. Eight-year-old Bud was responsible for delivering groceries by bike to nearby homes.

One day on his rounds, he was greeted by joy and tears as he dropped off a family's box of groceries. The frail children immediately began devouring the fruit. Young Bud left with a smile.

Returning home, he learned from his father that he had delivered the box to the wrong house. As the real customers had already paid and food stores were low on merchandise, Bud was forced to return and take the food back from the hungry family.

Later in life, Bud remembered feeling powerless that day to alleviate the hunger of those neighbors. He vowed that, when he grew up,

Bud Vogel *(right)* with his brother Joe in front of the family general store. Bud made his food deliveries on his bike.

he would do something to help the hungry of the Midwest.

"His experiences as a child, with the stark face of hunger all around, impacted and informed the rest of his life as he dedicated himself to

"WE NEED TO REMEMBER THAT THE FOODBANK'S CONSTITUENCY ARE THE POOR AND NEEDY THAT WE SERVE ON A DAILY BASIS."

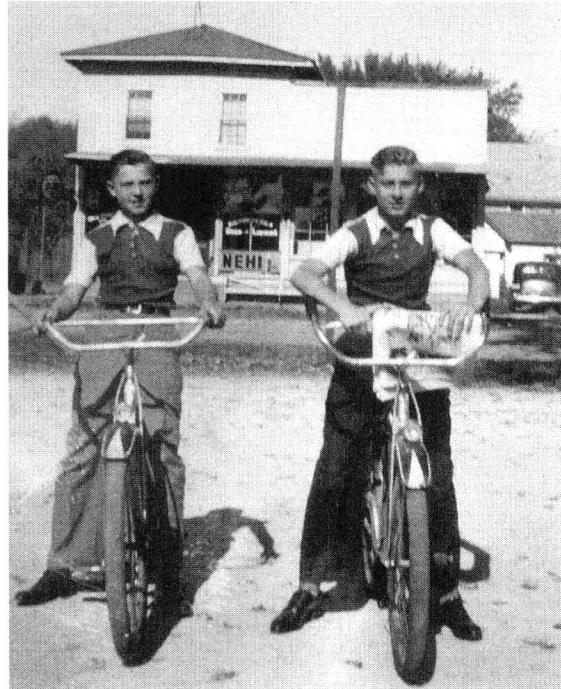

battling hunger," says his son Pete Vogel.

In 1982, Bud helped found the River Bend Foodbank, now located in Davenport, Iowa, and served as its chairman for 30 years. He also ran the St. Mary's Food Pantry at his local church, personally stocking shelves and handing food to the hungry each week.

Guided by his childhood experiences and his Catholic faith, Bud always strove to put himself in the shoes of the people he served.

"We need to remember that the Foodbank's constituency are the poor and needy that we serve on a daily basis," Bud wrote. "Let their plight guide and shape our commitment."

A deeply humble man with a quiet demeanor and warm smile, Bud deflected recognition for his work, instead encouraging his neighbors to focus on the hungry. His efforts paid off with the steady expansion of the River Bend Foodbank, which now distributes 8 million

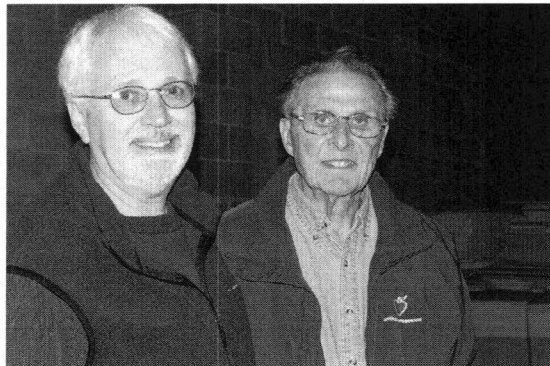

Bud Vogel, *right,* with Tom Laughlin, director of the River Bend Foodbank.

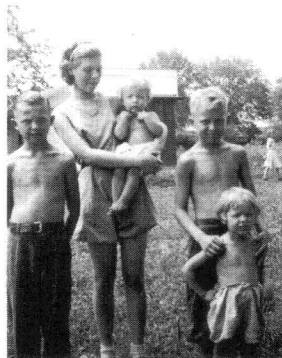

Bud Vogel *(fourth from the left)* as a boy with his siblings in Andalusia, Illinois, during the Great Depression. Writer Rachel Vogel Quinn's dad jokingly calls this the "Joad family photo," in reference to *The Grapes of Wrath.*

pounds of food annually to the needy in the Quad Cities and surrounding areas.

At the recent grand opening of the Foodbank's new 60,000-square-foot warehouse in Davenport, many commented that he was the heart and soul of the organization.

Bud passed away in March of 2013 after 30 years of serving the hungry and the hopeless. An inspiration for many in the area, Bud began his vocation by stocking shelves—and ended up nourishing lives.

HOW ARE *YOU* INSPIRED TO HELP THE HUNGRY? Share your story on the Hope for the Hungry Facebook page at **www.facebook.com/pages/ Hope-For-The-Hungry**.

15 Things You Can Do in the Next Hour

Still not sure how to help the hungry? Choose one of the following and make a start today!

1. Call your local food pantry and sign up to volunteer.

2. Search your own kitchen pantry for donation items.

3. Order seeds to start a small donation garden in your parking strip or backyard.

4. Buy groceries for a neighbor in need, or offer to take a homebound neighbor to the grocery store.

5. Sign up to drive for an organization that delivers meals to the elderly and homebound.

6. Schedule a time to speak to your congregation or service club about hunger in your community.

7. Make a post on social media to find out if any of your connections are involved in alleviating hunger. Ask how you can help.

8. Buy extra produce at the grocery store or farmer's market and take it to a food pantry.

9. Write a check to a worthy organization.

10. Gather up unused garden tools to take to a donation garden.

11. Call the principal at your local school to see if there are programs for food-insecure children. Ask how you can help.

12. Call your town or city council to find out how hunger is being addressed in your community.

13. Visit **iowahungerdirectory.org** to find organizations involved in alleviating hunger across Iowa.

14. Think about skills you could share, such as canning and preserving, gardening or cooking on a budget. Talk to your church or service club about utilizing or teaching what you know.

15. Share what you've learned in this resource guide with your family and friends!

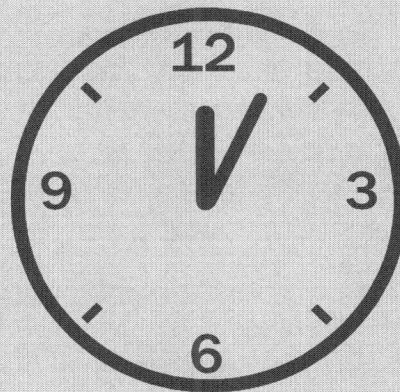

Discussion Questions

For use in your home, school, church, business or service organization, here are questions about each section of the Resource Guide *to inspire conversation and action.*

According to Reverend Diana Sickles, founder of the Hope for the Hungry conferences and the Coalition in Support of Hungry Children, the first four questions to ask yourself are:

- What is already being done here?
- How can I help?
- What isn't being done that needs to be?
- What can I do about it?

Keep those questions in mind as you discuss each section of this *Resource Guide* in more detail.

HUNGER AND NUTRITION

- Dr. David Spreadbury describes the many ways poor nutrition affects children. What's being done in your community to ensure proper nutrition for kids?
- Hunger—or malnutrition—often appears as obesity. Does this change your understanding of the hunger issue? In what way?
- Are healthy, affordable foods available in your community? If not, how could you improve access to them?
- In your own family, what's one small change you could make to eat more healthfully?
- Do you have a cooking skill or healthy recipe that you could share with food-insecure families?
- Are you involved in community organizations or clubs where food is served at gatherings? If so, how could you introduce healthier offerings at those gatherings?
- Childhood hunger has long-term consequences on our nation's health care costs. Weigh the cost effectiveness of these two options: using dollars and time now to alleviate food insecurity or paying for health costs down the road.
- Do the schools in your community participate in the national BackPack Program? If not, how could you help initiate one?
- Are there other ways you can help provide meals or groceries to food-insecure families during the weekend, when children may be going without proper nutrition?
- Is there a need for a high school food pantry in your community? Who could you work with to identify the need and launch a pantry program?
- Do you have food pantries in your area? If so, what items do they need most? What are their biggest challenges? Could you and a friend or family member volunteer?
- Are there children or adults falling through the gaps in the food distribution system in your community? How can you identify them?
- Are there other ways you could help raise

awareness about healthy food choices in your family, school, business, church or organization?

THE FACE OF HUNGER

- Do you have positive or negative perceptions about SNAP (also known as food stamps)? Why?

- Does Matt Russell's viewpoint about SNAP change your perceptions in any way?

- What do you think would happen to families who are food-insecure if the SNAP program weren't available?

- Do any of the facts about SNAP surprise you? If so, which ones? Why?

- Could grocery store tours be effective in your community?

- How could you identify parents who could benefit from the tours?

- What other forms of education do you think would help parents in food-insecure households?

- Does it surprise you that most food-insecure heads of household are employed?

- How might your own financial situation be affected if you got divorced, lost your spouse or job, or had a medical crisis?

- Does hunger in America affect hunger in other parts of the world? In what ways?

- Are there opportunities in your community to partner with corporations, churches or schools to use their land for donation gardens?

- Do you have a garden in your backyard? What do you do with the excess? Have you thought about growing an extra row for the hungry?

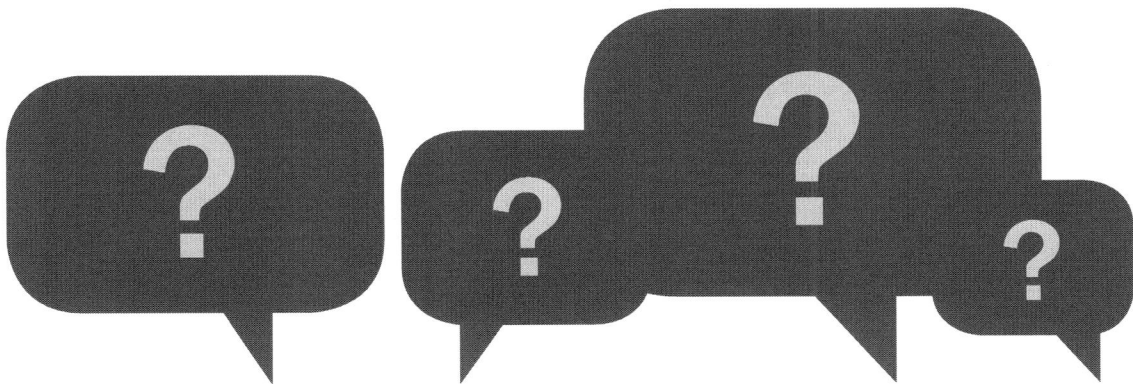

- Do you know veterans in your community who are food-insecure?

- If so, what are the realities of their financial situation? Do they receive VA benefits? Are they enrolled in SNAP?

- Does your place of business hire veterans?

- What could you, your church or your service organization do to reach out to vets?

- The Zestos program in northwest Iowa truly is a grassroots organization, starting from one family's desire to feed the hungry. Is there one thing you feel called to do?

THE ABCS OF ALLEVIATING HUNGER

- Many schools have classroom gardens and some kind of cooking/nutrition program. What's going on in your local schools about food and nutrition?

- Is it important for children to learn about food and where it comes from? Why or why not?

- Could your community provide an after-school nutrition program similar to the ASAP Culinary Arts Studio?

- Kids who help prepare foods show a greater willingness to try and enjoy vegetables. How could you put this to work in your family, church or youth group?

- Does your local high school have a food drive?

If not, how could you help start one? If it does, how could you increase awareness about it?

- Does your place of business donate food or volunteer hours to local food pantries or gardens? If not, how could you introduce this into your company's culture?

- Are your local schools engaged in the Farm to School program? How could the program benefit schoolchildren in your area? How could it be of help to the farmers?

RESCUING FOOD AND LAND

- How much food goes to waste in your home? How about in local businesses, restaurants and stores?

- What would it take in your community to establish a food rescue program? Who could the food be distributed to?

- As you go through your day, look at underutilized land in your area. Are there plots of land—like parking strips—that could be used to grow food?

- In addition to feeding the hungry, why does it make sense to utilize food, land—even deer—so they don't go to waste?

- In what ways can feeding the hungry help the people who donate the food? Are there other populations—like prisoners or refugees—who could benefit from getting involved in alleviating hunger?

- What corporations or foundations could you reach out to as a way of obtaining donations or sponsorships for worthy organizations or programs?

BRINGING IT ALL TOGETHER

- Many people who work to help the hungry are motivated by their faith. What motivates you to serve?

- What do you think of utilizing church land for donation gardens? What would be the biggest hurdles in starting such a garden, and how could those hurdles be overcome?

- Are there refugees from other countries in your community? Take time to talk with them about gardening. What did they grow in their homeland? What kind of relationship do they have with the land?

- Who are the stakeholders in your community? Who are the influencers who could help address hunger as part of a larger mission for a healthy community?

- What legacy do you want to leave? How could helping to alleviate hunger be part of that legacy?

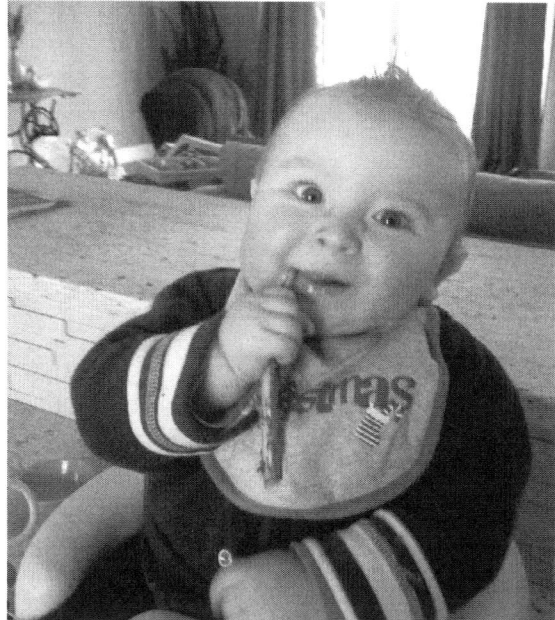

Need a reminder of why these questions matter? Here's Louie Bergquist of Nevada, Iowa, eating kale at an early age. What if every child could have this kind of health and vitality from proper nourishment?

Get involved, and you can help make it happen!

Thank You

This book would not have been possible without the financial support of donors who believe in a world without hunger. In contributing their dollars to this *Resource Guide*, they've helped alleviate food insecurity and built a stronger platform of positive change.

Platinum
Phil and Diana Sickles

Gold
Steve and Diane Harms
Mary Kay Riley
Bob and Sue Simons

Silver
Coalition in Support of Hungry Children
Hy-Vee, Inc.
Traditions Children's Center II, Inc.

Benefactor
Chuck and Regina Frevert
Riley Family Fund, Greater Des Moines
   Community Foundation
Neil and Debra Salowitz

Partner
Norm and Donna Barnes
Phil and Becky Bryant
Owen Christoferson
Ruth H. Cooperrider
Richard and Bonnie Ekse
Russell, Jr. and Lucile Johnson
Pat and Tricia Owens

Mark and Janet Rosenbury
Jean Rothfusz
Chuck and Pam Schoffner
Bob and Pat Schroeder
Sally Simmel
Aaron and Jan Stegeman

Supporter
Anonymous
Don and Carolyn Beck
Erin Bergquist
Randy L. Clarke
Ken Cheyne
James and Celeste Egger
Tracy Fiese and Marla Downey
Kathleen Frevert and Howard Levenson
Marshall and Jerry Grabau
Joie Gronert
Steve and Cheryl Hamilton
Norma Hirsch
John and Karol Joenks
Dan and Julie Kaercher
Dean and Marie Kayser
Kent and Karen Klopfenstein
Keith and Diane Krell
Phil and Judy Latessa
Lioness Club of Urbandale

Rich and Sue Mandt
Robert and Helen McAfoos
Vince and Marva McCarty
Ray and Susan Meylor
Eleanor Monahan
Vernon and Joyce Naffier
Carla Peterman
Jim and Connie Ridge
Jeff and Susan Rissman
Sharpe Family Dentistry, P.C.
Bob and Becky Shaw
Vaun and Marian Sprecher
Kelly and Angela Tagtow
Jeff and Connie Ryan Terrell
Margaret Weiner
W.I.L.P.F.
Irving and Diane Wolfe
Women of the Evangelical Lutheran
    Church in America, Cluster 9
Roland and Barbara Zimany

Friend

Craig and Linda Ackarman
Jeff and Mary Ellen Anderson
Bob Andrlik
Kent and Jeannette Babcock
Jean Boomershine
Joyce Coon
Brena Corona
Jim and Mary Covey
Denise Crawford
Gloria Criswell
Clint and Carole Curtis

Helen Dagley
Vi Darsee
Peter and Carol Dittmer
DeVonne Douglas
Neal and Sheryl Feuerhelm
Ellen Fisher
Bob and Phyllis Gale
Mike Gaul and Ann Taylor
Marilyn Gibbs
Diane Glass
foodandyou/Linda Gobberdiel
Gayle Goodale
Bonnie Green
Kris and Kathy Gregersen
Kay Grother
Terry and Ginny Hancock
George and Janet Hanusa
Heads Up
Ed and Helen Heusinkveld
Harry and Starr Hinrichs
Larry and Karen Hoier
Doug and Randi Holmgren
Julie Honsey
Roger and Sue Hudson
Dick and Carolyn Hutton
Jane Ibsen
Bob and Marilynn Johnson
Doug and Stephanie Johnson
Don and Truly Judisch
Lisa Kilmer
Greg and Susan Klein
Dennis and Karen Kral
Curt and Patty Lack

Bob and Pam Larson
John Leiendecker and Linda Vanderloo
Jean LemMon
Paul and Anita Lindstrom
Chip and Julie Lowe
Jim and Ruth Lundeen
David Maxey
Mary Mincer and Roger Hansen
Bob Mitchell and Jan Burch
Nancy Mohlis
Lee and Ginny Molgaard
Ed and Vi Munsch
Craig and Shaunda Murphy
Ron and Carolyn Nielsen
Lance and Debbie Noe
Jim and Shelley Noyce
Michael and Gail Pace
William and Regina Pace
Don and Linda Palmer
Jim and Jane Patten
Randy and Ginny Pauling
Roger and Susan Petersen
Elise Pohl
Susan Pohl
Katherine G. Rovane
Steve and Marlys Ruth
Pat and Mary Ryan
Lowell and Rita Samuelson
Bill and Karen Schoenenberger
Dal Schroeder
Yogesh Shah
Ed and Mary Slattery
Tom and Barb Sletto

Larry and Ruth Smith
Olga Sparks
Bob and Terri Speirs
Herb and Joan Strentz
LeAnn Stubbs
Sara Sutton
Ron Taylor
Willa J. Tharp
Bill and Bonnie Theisen
Harold and Virginia Varce
Joel Waymire
Fred and Donna Wessendorf
Nicky Wynne

Acknowledgments

This *Resource Guide* and its companion DVD would not have been possible without the help of countless people who believed in and supported this project with their information, their time and their dollars. We are indebted to:

The leadership team of the Coalition in Support of Hungry Children for their help in organizing and promoting the Hope for the Hungry conference, which served as the catalyst for this project.

Pam Schoffner, communications consultant and owner of P.S. Writes, who provided invaluable experience in fund-raising, marketing and promotion.

Larrison Seidle, the creative mind behind the design of this *Resource Guide*, for his sheer determination despite sometimes daunting challenges.

Mary Heaton, professional proofreader, for her eagle eyes and attention to detail.

The Iowa Food Systems Council, for their leadership and education in supporting healthy communities, and for serving as the fiscal agent for this project.

Phil Sickles, whose rare blend of humor, business acumen and deep concern for others offered balance and wisdom throughout the process.

And to Diana Sickles, founder of the Coalition in Support of Hungry Children, whose passion for feeding the hungry has impacted more lives than she will ever know.

We thank them all.